31 MAKEUP ESSENTIALS
Unlock Your Ultimate Beauty Kit

AMITA GOEL

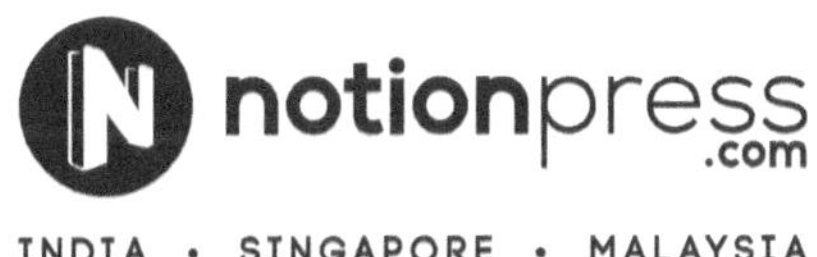

INDIA · SINGAPORE · MALAYSIA

ISBN
Paperback 979-8-89632-335-8
Hardcase 979-8-89777-879-9

Contents

The Inspiration

For as long as I can remember, I dreamed of writing a book. But as a homemaker, self-doubt crept in, whispering that I wasn't enough. So, instead, I wanted my children—bright and full of potential—to be the ones to write the book I could not. Like any typical Asian mum, I nudged, encouraged, and pushed them to achieve greatness each day.

However, I soon realised that their dreams were different from mine. They had their own goals, aspirations, and life challenges to face. One day, they sat me down and said, "Mum, we're already swamped. There's no time to write a book."

That moment was bittersweet. Once again, I questioned myself: Was I being too demanding? But then came a spark of clarity. **What if I wrote the book myself?** What if, by doing so, I could inspire them to take on even bigger challenges in life? After all, monkey see, monkey do.

Over the years, several people suggested I write about my experiences— how I managed to stay resourceful while navigating life with a husband whose job required relocations. Though I often dismissed the idea, taking things at face value, it lingered in the back of my mind. But it wasn't until my pageant journey that I truly understood my purpose. I wanted to write more about **my path towards living a medicine-free life**.

As I began writing, another idea tugged at me—what about chronicling my pageant journey? And then, as I explored even further, makeup—a crucial part of that journey—demanded my attention. The struggle to achieve the perfect look and master those necessary touch-ups was real. I bought endless products based on advice from makeup enthusiasts and artists without fully understanding their use.

But in every struggle, I believe there's an idea waiting to emerge if only we pay attention. After a year of having my makeup done by various artists for fashion shows and photoshoots, I decided to learn the craft, get certified as a makeup artist, and even become an International Airbrush Makeup Artist. Finally, I understood how to choose and use the products and tools that truly suited me.

This book is born from my love for makeup and the countless trials and errors I faced. It's meant to be a guide—a companion for anyone planning to navigate the overwhelming world of makeup products and tools. I hope it simplifies your makeup purchase journey and inspires you to embrace your creativity, just as I have.

Gratitude

There are people in our lives who believe in us even when we doubt ourselves, and their unwavering faith becomes the light that guides us forward. For me, my daughter, Ruhi Kumar, is one of those people—an endless fountain of encouragement, empowerment, and love. Even when I faltered, her belief in me gave me the strength to pursue dreams I once thought were beyond my reach. To Ruhi, I owe my deepest gratitude. She's a constant source of support and a reminder of why it's essential to keep pushing forward, even when self-doubt looms.

I also extend my heartfelt thanks to Bhumika Bahl, an extraordinary makeup educator. I have always believed that growth doesn't come from simply meeting the best people but from crossing paths with the right ones. Bhumika is undoubtedly one of those rare individuals whose kindness and generosity know no bounds. She is a giver, a nurturer, someone who nourishes the souls of those around her. Her vision goes beyond makeup—uplifting her learners, empowering them with new skills, and helping them achieve personal growth and financial independence.

Bhumika's passion for life and insightful lessons about the world resonates deeply with me. She doesn't just teach makeup; she imparts wisdom about navigating the broader challenges of life. Her warmth, sincerity, and genuine desire to see others succeed have impacted me. I had the privilege of learning closely under her guidance. In every interaction, her selfless support and inspiring gestures shone through. Her ability to uplift and empower others is more than a profession; it's her calling. I am incredibly grateful for her presence in my life as she inspires me and many others to grow, evolve, and achieve our fullest potential.

I would also like to thank Tejasvi Kaul, my son's friend and trained Bharatnatyam dancer. With her keen eye for performance makeup, she managed to find time from her busy corporate schedule to sit with me to read this book before its submission to the publishing house. Her honest feedback gave me the confidence to submit my work on time without any delay.

Introduction: My Story

Though I spent much of my life hidden behind oversized clothes and kept grooming at arm's length, my love for makeup never truly faded. This love, along with my passion for fashion, was reignited during my pageant journey – a journey that would change my life forever.

After more than 30 years of marriage, I finally had the chance to pursue a childhood dream: participating in a beauty pageant. Growing up, I had always admired the grace and confidence of pageant contestants, but I never imagined it could be my reality. That door was opened for me by my son, who, in our typically patriarchal family setup, gave me the support I needed to take that leap. His faith in me was extraordinary and unexpected, especially when I grappled with self-doubt. He encouraged me to work on myself, just as the younger contestants are required to do, reminding me that it's never too late to chase your dreams.

It was in June 2023 when my mentor, Anjali Raut, encouraged me to enter a pageant for women in my age group—an opportunity I hadn't even known was possible. After passing the auditions, I embarked on a journey filled with firsts, exploring aspects of beauty, fashion, and self-expression that my heart had always longed for but had never pursued.

This experience felt like a stroke of luck, but in my heart, I knew it was meant to be. It deepened my belief that dreams are gifts from God. When we listen to the quiet call of our soul and pursue our true desires, the journey—no matter how challenging—brings a sense of bliss. It is a calling.

My dream journey culminated in a national victory, winning the prestigious **Elite Queen Of The World India** title. Under the able guidance of Urmimala Boruah, CEO of UMB Pageants, this achievement propelled me further, giving me the honour of representing India on the international stage in April 2024, where I secured the 1st runner-up position, Elite Queen Of The World.

Throughout this transformative experience, I came to understand that looking good on the outside—through makeup and fashion—is just as important as taking care of the inside for healthy, glowing skin, as it is the foundation of true beauty. This realisation has become a cornerstone of my approach to makeup and self-care.

How I Learned About Makeup

We were expected to be as presentable as seasoned contestants during pageant training. Like me, most of the girls were still learning, so the focus was on the effort everyone put into their transformation. Some girls had prior experience with makeup or pageantry, but for me, everything was new—from wearing fitted clothes to confidently donning off-shoulder dresses and elegant gowns. Despite my lack of experience, I never felt out of place. My enthusiasm to make the most of this opportunity kept me moving forward. The learning environment was warm and welcoming at Cocoaberry and the girls—most of whom were less than half my age—were sweet and helpful. Their youthful energy matched my eagerness to absorb everything, and I thoroughly enjoyed their company.

Pageant life, though, is more than just walking gracefully or smiling on cue. It's about photo shoots, high-definition images, making reels, and posting on social media, all of which demand a constantly polished look. That's when makeup becomes not just an accessory but a necessity. I quickly realised that, like every other pageant aspect, I had to master makeup. For nearly a year, I relied on professional makeup artists as I progressed from the national platform to the international stage. And while they worked wonders, the thought that haunted me was this: I needed an artist every time I faced a camera. The camera tells no lies. It captures every flaw, every shadow, and I knew I had to look my best in every frame. But there was a nagging thought—I didn't have the skills to do this alone.

That's when I began searching for someone to teach me this fundamental art. I didn't just want the best; I needed the right person to guide me. As I explored my options, an AI algorithm suggested Bhumika Bahl. When I discovered her, I was convinced she was the educator I needed. She not only had the skills but also the generosity to share her knowledge.

Brushes and sponges became my tools, my face became my canvas, and my hands learned through trial and error. After a shower, giving myself a quick makeup session became something I started to enjoy. It was me time—a fun, creative escape. With her keen eye, my daughter would inspect my efforts over WhatsApp calls, offering feedback. My husband, however, was not as interested. For him, makeup meant nothing; he was happy with how I looked in my natural state—carelessly made hair, pyjamas, and all. My son was more indifferent, adopting the attitude of "Do what makes you happy." If I pressed him for feedback, his response was always, "You're looking nice."

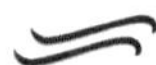

Why I Wrote This Book

Early in my pageant journey, I realised that mastering makeup wasn't just an option but a necessity. Every detail counted, and I wanted to be in control of my appearance, owning each look with confidence. Despite taking several personal makeup sessions with various artists, I craved more. I didn't just want fragmented knowledge—I needed a well-structured, thoughtfully curated programme that would teach me the art of makeup and help me navigate the overwhelming choices available in the beauty world. I was searching for a mentor, not just someone skilled but someone who could guide me with expertise, patience, and care. And then, as if fate were listening, I discovered Bhumika Bahl. Her passion, her talent, and her thoughtful approach were exactly what I had been searching for. She wasn't just a makeup educator—she was the guide I needed.

There's plenty of information about makeup on social media - from influencers to beauty brands, the flood of tutorials and recommendations can leave you more confused than empowered. The beauty industry is booming, with new products hitting the shelves almost daily. Yet, with so many options, the question remains—how do you know what's right for you? When I started, my makeup vanity was filled with products I didn't know how or when to use. The overwhelming number of brushes, kits, and palettes felt more like a puzzle than a toolbox.

For most makeup enthusiasts, especially those just starting out, navigating this world can be daunting. As a beginner, I remember trying to keep up with the list of products required for my classes. To avoid embarrassment, I bought everything on the list—often in large quantities—to find myself using only a handful. Even a year later, many of those products remain untouched. Investing in quality makeup can be worthwhile, but it's equally important to know **how much is too much and how much is just enough.**

For many of us, makeup is not just about looking good; it's an expression of who we are. But it also comes with a cost that reflects the hard-earned money we, or someone close to us, put into building that vanity. Understanding our products, knowing how to use them, and choosing the right tools to achieve our desired looks are essential. Otherwise, we risk wasting our money and the opportunity to enhance our natural beauty effectively.

That's why I wrote this book. I want to share my journey, my lessons, and my insights to help others avoid the mistakes I made. I wish this book empowers my readers to make informed decisions about their makeup, to understand what they truly need, and to master the art of makeup in a way that complements their unique beauty. This book is my way of helping you navigate the overwhelming world of beauty products with confidence and clarity so you can create the looks you've always dreamed of—without the clutter.

Why This Book Will Benefit You

In my journey, both as a homemaker and during my pageant experiences, I have had the privilege of meeting many remarkable women. Like so many of us, these women share a passion for beauty and an undeniable attraction to the ever-growing world of cosmetics. For some, walking into a store and seeing a new product on the shelf is a guilty pleasure they cannot resist. With the increasing number of salons, makeup services, and countless beauty brands vying for attention, our wallets often speak louder than our needs.

Many of us can relate to the desire to look beautiful, and the beauty industry has expanded immensely to cater to those desires, particularly for women. While I hope this book will help many, my primary focus is on homemakers above 50 and the next generation, Generation Alpha.

Through my own experiences, I have learned the importance and power of authenticity. We live in a world full of beauty products and trends, but it's important to find clarity in our choices: the choices we make versus the ones we truly want to make. This book will take you on a journey of self-reflection, guiding you to think about the looks you want to create and the image you wish to project. It's not just about looking good but about ensuring that your appearance truly reflects who you are inside—and how you want the world to perceive you.

As I write each chapter, I am genuinely excited about how this book will be received. My goal is to help you make sense of the overwhelming beauty market, guiding you towards the right products and tools so that when you step out to make a purchase, you do so confidently. This book is my sincere effort to save you time and money while helping you avoid wasteful purchases.

In addition to this, I highly recommend investing in good-quality training, whether through a professional academy or personal grooming sessions. Learning this art is a way to express your creativity every day, and it can also empower you to help others feel more confident in their own skin. If I had to name this training and skill, I would call it '**Learn and Earn**.' The best thing about quality makeup training is that you can start earning immediately after learning. This book is not just about looking beautiful—it's about embracing the power that comes with knowing how to enhance your beauty and share that confidence with those around you.

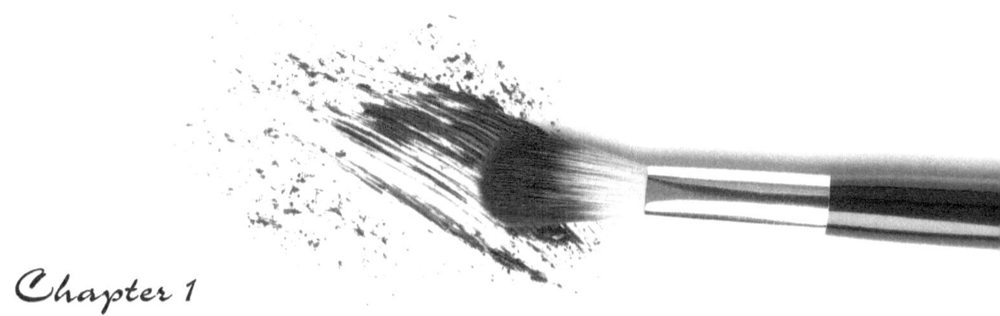

Chapter 1

Approach to Makeup

During my pageant journey, I discovered something truly transformative: the power of grooming. Makeup and self-care became more than just daily routines – they became acts of self-love, a way to enhance my appearance and confidence. It became clear that beauty isn't just about the products we use; it's about how those products make us feel.

As I ventured deeper into the world of makeup, I noticed that people approach it in three distinct ways:

- **The Minimalists** are drawn to simplicity. A swipe of kajal, a touch of lipstick—this is all it takes for them to feel beautiful. Their mantra is *"less is more,"* and their effortless routines exude a refreshing and inspiring charm. I used to be one of them, content with just the basics.

- **The Occasionals** bring out their makeup for special moments. BB or CC cream, a hint of colour here and there—they savour the process of enhancing their appearance without making it a daily ritual. For them, makeup is a celebration, a way to highlight the importance of an event. This was my approach when I was younger, and it still makes me smile when I think about it.

- **Enthusiasts** are those who have mastered the art of makeup. Their flawless looks leave us both in awe and, sometimes, a bit intimidated. We admire their skill, though we might wonder if they take it too far. Regardless, their dedication is undeniable.

I began as a Minimalist, with a routine that involved little more than kajal and my favourite lipstick. However, I often found myself disheartened when my kajal would smudge by the end of the day. In 2013, I developed dry eyes, which made wearing kajal uncomfortable. As my doctor advised me to avoid applying it on my waterline, I was pushed to find alternative makeup methods. I turned to blush and uncovered new ways to express my love for makeup. However, my passion for it didn't fully blossom until my national win as Elite Queen Of The World India in 2023.

When I was young, there was no social media coaching or YouTube tutorials to guide me, so I relied solely on my instincts. I focused on enhancing my natural beauty, not covering it up, and this journey became a beautiful process of self-discovery. I learned that grooming is not just about looking good – it's about embracing individuality and feeling confident in your skin.

When I decided to write this book, it came from a simple wish: to help others avoid the struggles I faced when trying to find the right beauty products. As a mother, I often thought about what advice I would give my daughter as she navigates the endless beauty options. I didn't want her to feel overwhelmed.

I remembered the countless hours I spent experimenting with products, searching for what worked best. I sought expert advice, yet it often felt like piecing together a puzzle. Many kept their beauty secrets close, and I was left to figure things out through trial and error. Through this process, I realised that no one should have to go through this alone.

That's why I created this book – to be a companion on your beauty journey. It's here to help you curate a personalised list of must-have products tailored to your needs. I want this book to be a warm, guiding hand, especially for those stepping into the world of makeup for the first time, like teenagers finding their identity or homemakers juggling endless responsibilities while trying to find time for themselves.

With this book, I hope you feel empowered to make choices that reflect your true beauty. Together, we'll turn what can feel like an overwhelming task into an exciting adventure. Let's embrace the journey of self-discovery, *one product at a time.*

In today's world, learning makeup has never been more accessible. With the wealth of online tutorials and resources, the beauty landscape is accessible to everyone. We only need to find our calling, practice what we've learned, and share our knowledge with others who seek to grow. Embrace the journey of learning makeup—it's not just about looking beautiful; it's about feeling confident and empowered.

Makeup is a powerful tool that celebrates the unique beauty within each of us. *When we look beautiful, we feel beautiful, and that feeling radiates confidence.* This book is my honest effort to help you navigate the beauty world, feel good in your skin, and create a visual presence that reflects the best version of yourself.

Like ghee hidden in butter or butter unseen in milk, our most potent beauty lies within us. By learning a bit of grooming, we can bring forth our best selves to live our dreams and inspire those around us.

So, let's create a beautiful you that reflects your personality and style, with makeup as your tool for daily self-expression. As you play with products and colours, *you'll unleash the creativity waiting to shine, just like your dreams.*

My Dream

As a young girl, I was captivated by the beauty world—fine clothes, makeup, hair, and trendy jewellery. I dreamed of being a fashion designer, envisioning a life filled with creativity and elegance. Back then, terms like "image consultant" didn't exist, but looking back, I realise that's exactly what I wanted to be. As I looked in the mirror each morning, I saw a canvas—God's beautiful creation. I expressed my gratitude by keeping it clean and well-kept and adding little touches of decoration, just like adorning a temple. To me, honouring my body is akin to decorating a deity, an act of respect and love.

But life had other plans. I was born into a conservative family with an orthodox father who valued simplicity above all else. He never allowed me to experiment with fashion or makeup, and he thought I was brimming with ideas and creative energy, so I could not follow my heart. Yet, I never rebelled. My childhood was full of love and laughter, and my parents' immense care and protection made it hard for me to go against their wishes. To them, simplicity was the essence of beauty, and in their eyes, I was already their princess, the most precious and beautiful baby girl.

Marriage brought a continuation of this life. My husband, a true gentleman, loved me deeply and took exceptional care of me. He complimented me in the simplest of attires, and I, once again, found myself holding back my personal desires to keep peace and harmony. His happiness became my priority, and I never felt the heart to challenge his preferences. As a devoted wife and homemaker, life was fulfilling in many ways, but my dreams—those creative desires—remained tucked away, quietly waiting.

Then, something unusual happened after more than 30 years of marriage. After dedicating myself to my family, children, and home, an unexpected opportunity arose. The world of beauty pageants opened before me, feeling like a divine sign. This was my calling, something I had been waiting for all along. With God's grace and the encouragement of my loved ones, I ventured into this new world with all my heart. Pageantry became the key that unlocked the part of me that had been dormant for so long.

Winning the national pageant was not just a victory but an awakening. It empowered me in ways I had never imagined. For the first time, I truly felt in charge of my life. I realised that our dreams are not meant to be hidden, wrapped away in some forgotten corner of our hearts. They are gifts waiting to be found, unwrapped, and shared with the world. Pageantry gave me the courage to bring my dreams into the light and to show the world who I truly am.

Now, the dream of sharing what I have learned with others has given rise to this book. I am pouring my heart into sharing my experience as a guide to makeup and as a tool to empower women, especially homemakers and the younger generation. It's an effort to inspire every woman to feel confident, emboldened, and in control of her beauty choices. I believe this book has the potential to be a trusted ally, helping women cross-check their makeup essentials and feel beautiful every day.

Take a Breath & Reflect: The Beauty in Choices

Before we dive in, let's slow down for a moment. Find a comfy seat, close your eyes, and relax. Let your body soften—unclench your jaw, release your tongue, and ease your mind. Now, reflect:

> *"Ever found yourself drowning in a sea of makeup products, unsure where to begin? I've been there too! But don't worry, this book is your shortcut to mastering the essentials—let's be honest, who's got the time (or patience) to test 100 different foundations?"*

Now, take a minute to really think about the following questions. Re-read them if necessary. Let your mind wander, and pay close attention to your thoughts.

1. **How do you feel about yourself right now?** Do you feel beautiful? Confident? Or is there a little whisper of self-doubt?
2. **What if I told you that spending just 20 minutes on yourself each day could boost your look and make you feel more presentable and polished?** How would that change how you feel or impact your life, career, or relationships?

If you're nodding along, thinking, *"Yes, that's exactly what I need,"* guess what? This book is for you. Think of it as your perfect coffee table companion, shopping list guide, or light read with serious potential to help elevate your presence.

A Beauty Revolution That Starts with You

Yes, we've got beauty parlours on every street corner and fancy beauty academies around every bend, ready to boost your confidence and make you feel like a star. But imagine if you could do it yourself. Imagine having the skills to bring out your best *on your own*. I am not just a makeup artist; I see myself as your personal beauty educator, a guide who helps you make the right choices to curate a beauty kit that reflects your personal style.

Think of it like a job interview. Imagine two candidates—both equally qualified, equally brilliant, and equally beautiful. But one of them took that extra step, adding a little polish to their appearance, amplifying their best features. Which one do you think gets chosen?

Teenagers & Timeless Queens

Working with teenagers is especially close to my heart because I believe learning to feel beautiful and confident sets you up for success. But you know who else I am here for? Women over 50—especially homemakers. Because I understand where they come from. I have walked that road myself, and my heart reaches out to those who feel like the doors of opportunity never opened. Together, we'll unlock those doors and take steps towards becoming the best version of ourself—version 2.0.

This isn't just a journey of makeup—it's an endeavour to become more confident, inspired, and happier. I am here to guide and support you every step of the way.

CTM – Your Skincare Essentials

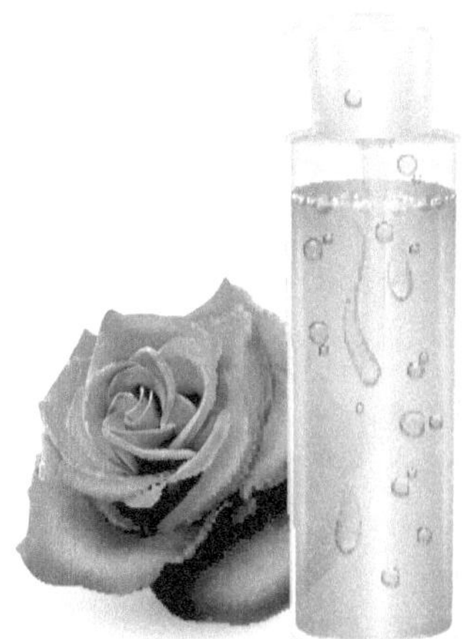

If you're a makeup lover, you've probably heard of CTM: Cleansing, Toning, and Moisturising. It's the step-by-step skincare routine we all need, whether we plan to wear makeup or not. CTM is your skin's daily dose of love—morning and night.

But since the lockdown, there's an extra step we cannot forget—SCTM. Yes, **sanitisation** has become essential to our skincare routine, especially before touching our face or letting someone else (like a makeup artist) do so. Don't forget to wash your hands if you're doing your own skincare or makeup!

Before We Start: Know Your Skin

Before diving into your CTM routine, take a moment to really know your skin. After all, skin is our largest organ, and it absorbs everything it touches through its pores.

Activity Time!

Grab a mirror and carefully observe your skin. Is it dry, oily, combination, or sensitive? How did you figure this out? Was it something you read, or did someone else tell you? Have you become aware through your own careful observation?

Skin Types & How to Care for Them

Let's break down the basics based on my experiences. For scientific details, Google can be your best friend!

Dry Skin:

It often looks dull, and it may appear flaky during colder months. To check if your skin is dry, try this: softly scratch the surface of your skin with your nail. Does it leave a mark? If yes, you likely have dry skin.

- **Inner Care**: I have found that eating water-rich fruits and veggies does wonders. "Eat your water," as they say; nature has packed them with hydration and nutrients. Drink water when you're thirsty, but sip slowly, letting it swirl in your mouth before swallowing. This conscious hydration improved my skin texture and even lightened pigmentation!
- **Outer Care**: Keep your skin hydrated with moisturisers, creams, or oils.

Oily Skin:

Oily skin feels greasy and often looks shiny due to overactive sebaceous glands.

Outer Care: Cleanse gently twice a day to remove excess oil and dirt. Oily skin tends to attract dust, so keeping it clean is essential.

Combination Skin:

This skin type is dry on the cheeks and oily in the T-zone (forehead, nose, and chin). You'll usually notice the shine on the T-zone, especially in the mornings.

Outer Care: Use a gentle cleanser and a denser moisturiser on dry areas like the cheeks.

Sensitive Skin:

If your skin reacts easily, it's probably sensitive. But what's causing that sensitivity? Is it the sun, cosmetics, food, or something else? It's best to consult a dermatologist to get to the root of it.

Inner Care: The Key to Healthy Skin

From my experience, nature is our healer. If we pay attention to it, it will pay attention to us. Though I have mentioned how we can care for the skin externally, I believe inner care is more important for achieving healthy, balanced skin.

What we put inside our bodies is as important as what we apply outside. Nourish your body with ripe fruits and vegetables—eat them or drink fresh juices. Nature's food will help create balance within the body.

Morning Routine: CTMB (Cleanse, Tone, Moisturise, Balm)

After your shower, it's time to give your skin some love. Here's how I do it:

1. **Cleanse**: Use a gentle wipe or face wash to remove leftover grime. Your pores are open, so let's start fresh.
   - Dry Skin: Use a gentle cleanser that preserves natural oils.
   - Oily Skin: Cleanse to remove excess oil and dirt.
   - Combination Skin: Use a gentle cleanser to balance dry areas and oily patches.
   - Sensitive Skin: Use a non-irritating cleanser to protect the skin barrier.

2. **Toner**: Spritz your favourite toner to further hydrate and refresh your skin. I personally love rose-scented toners—it's like a mini spa moment and always brings a smile to my face.
   - Dry Skin/ Oily skin: Toners add an extra layer of hydration.
   - Combination Skin: Ensures balance between dry and oily areas.
   - Sensitive Skin: Use toners free from potential irritants to calm and soothe the skin.

3. **Moisturise**: This is where the magic happens. I used to apply a moisturiser with my palms, but professionals often use brushes. During my international pageant journey, I learned firsthand the importance of hydration when a makeup artist applied the same generous amount of moisturiser to both me (with dry-normal skin) and my daughter (with combination skin). That was my "aha" moment—hydrated skin makes all the difference!
   - Dry Skin: Locks in moisture and prevents dehydration.
   - Oily Skin: Use lightweight, oil-free moisturisers to hydrate without clogging pores.

Common mistake: Over-moisturising oily skin

- ▶ Combination Skin: Use a lighter moisturiser for oily areas and a denser one for dry patches.
- ▶ Sensitive Skin: Opt for fragrance-free, hypoallergenic moisturisers.

4. **Balm**: Don't forget the lips! Whether you like a tinted balm or something fragrance-free, keep your lips moisturised too.

Night Routine: RCTMB (Remove, Cleanse, Tone, Moisturise, Balm)

Before bed, follow these five steps to feel fresh, relaxed, and ready for a good night's sleep.

1. **Remove Makeup**: Never skip this step! I love using cold-pressed coconut oil to gently remove makeup. It's hydrating and doesn't strip the skin of moisture.
2. **Cleanse**: Once makeup is off, use a gentle face wash for an extra clean.
3. **Tone**: Spritz toner to close your pores and enjoy the soothing mist.
4. **Moisturise**: Apply 2-3 pumps of a moisturiser using a brush or fingertips and let it work its magic overnight.
5. **Balm**: Finish with lip balm to keep your lips soft and supple!

My Story: From Besan to Beauty

Growing up, I swore by natural ingredients—besan (gram flour), ground lentils, and fuller's earth (*multani mitti*) were my go-to cleansers instead of soap. However, as I entered the makeup world, I began to appreciate the importance of following a structured skincare routine in the correct order. Did I face any challenges?

Absolutely, pageant preparation pushed me out of my comfort zone and led to personal transformation. As I was exploring life, I encountered many new facets. I experienced and embraced them as an experiment to evolve into a new version of myself.

Nowadays, I use this routine when I wear makeup. Some days, I just let my skin breathe, free of products, especially when soaking in the morning sun, enjoying the fresh air, and reconnecting with nature.

Remember: Your skin is unique, and so is your journey. Whether you're a skincare newbie or a seasoned pro, it's all about finding what works best for you.

We have only one face, yet it often gets neglected in the hustle of life. Whether we are stay-at-home mums, college students, or corporate workers, we can still give our face the basic attention it needs to stay hydrated and look healthy. At the very least, this is the basic minimum we can do for our face.

"No matter where you are in your skincare journey, every step forward is progress!"

Reflection Time

Now that we've explored the essentials of CTMB, let's take a moment to reflect on them. Grab a pencil and write down your thoughts:

1. How does your current skincare routine look like compared to what you've learned here?
2. Think about the steps you're already taking and which ones you might miss.
3. What small changes would you like to improve your routine?
4. Sometimes, the little things make the most significant difference. What tweaks can help you get the most out of your skincare?

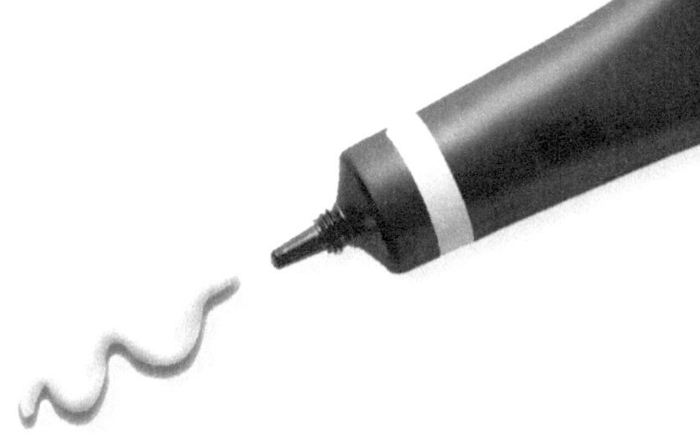

Chapter 3

Primer – The Essential Base for Flawless Makeup

While many professionals in the makeup industry refer to CTMP (cleaning, tone, moisturising, priming) as a routine, I want to separate "Priming" for those who may only choose to follow a skincare routine. However, primer is an essential product if you're applying makeup and want a flawless, long-lasting look.

What is Primer?

Primer is used to create a smooth, flawless base that enhances the overall look of your makeup. Applied before foundation, it improves the skin's appearance by minimising pores and creating a smooth surface. It acts as a barrier between your skin and makeup, ensuring that foundation, concealer, and other products glide on smoothly and blend seamlessly. Beyond blurring imperfections, primer helps even out your skin texture and prolongs the wear of your makeup.

Application Tips for a Smooth Base

After completing your CTM routine, apply a primer in small quantities, focusing on areas with enlarged pores or uneven texture. Use a brush or your fingertips; many professionals prefer using your fingers for better control. Be mindful not to overapply; too much primer can cause makeup to slide off. The goal is to create a smooth, even canvas for your foundation, allowing it to blend effortlessly.

Types of Primers

With so many primer options on the market—hydrating, mattifying, illuminating, and more—it can feel overwhelming. Here's a simple rule: choose based on your skin type.

- **For Dry Skin**: Hydrating primers add moisture and prevent the foundation from settling into dry patches.
- **For Oily Skin**: A mattifying primer controls shine and helps makeup last longer by minimising excess oil.
- **For Combination Skin**: Use a primer that balances dry and oily areas or select one labelled "for all skin types."
- **For Sensitive Skin**: Choose primers with calming ingredients that won't irritate your skin.

If you're unsure of your skin type, a safe choice is a primer labelled "suitable for all skin types."

My Realisations About Primers

I used to consider primer an extra, non-essential step reserved only for special occasions. But after realising how it prevents makeup from melting off in the heat or under stage lights, I now consider it essential—even for daily wear.

I suggest paying close attention to your makeup removal routine for those worried about primer clogging pores. Proper cleansing will keep your skin healthy and your pores clear.

Choosing the right ingredients based on your skin's needs can be a game-changer. Primer gives makeup something to adhere to, ensuring an even application. Think of your face as a blank canvas and primer as the smooth gesso layer an artist applies before starting their work of art.

Real-Life Situations Where Primer Saved the Day

One hot summer day in Delhi, I attended a victory party the UMB pageants team arranged after a historic win at the international platform in New York. The harsh sun of the month of May had me worried about my makeup melting off, but the makeup artist assured me that a good primer would prevent my foundation from separating. Despite the sweaty afternoon, my makeup remained intact. That day, I realised how crucial primer can be, especially in hot, humid conditions. It wasn't just about making my makeup last longer—it kept it fresh and flawless throughout the day.

Another personal mishap highlighted the importance of primer. On the day of my daughter's National Memory Championship in Hyderabad in October 2024, I skipped it and noticed uneven patches of foundation on her face a couple of hours later. It was a wake-up call. Since then, I have never skipped primer, especially when I need my makeup to look flawless for long periods.

Reflection: Primer as the Foundation of Makeup

Primer is like the foundation of a house. Without it, makeup crumbles and settles into imperfections, which means it looks patchy over time, depending on your skin.

Understanding your skin type and specific makeup needs can help you choose the right primer to enhance your look and ensure long-lasting, smooth results.

Reflection Exercise

This exercise will help you reflect on your skin type, needs, and preferences and guide you in choosing the best primer for your makeup routine.

1. **Identify Your Skin Type**: After cleansing your face, wait 30 minutes without applying any products. How does your skin feel?

    ► Tight or flaky: **Dry Skin**

    ► Shiny on the T-zone but normal elsewhere: **Combination Skin**

    ► Shiny all over: **Oily Skin**

    ► Easily irritated or sensitive: **Sensitive Skin**

2. **Which of the following is your biggest makeup concern?**

    ► Enlarged pores or uneven texture

    ► Makeup sliding off throughout the day

    ► Skin appearing too dry or dull

    ► Excess oil and shine

    ► Redness, discoloration, or hyperpigmentation

3. **Based on your skin type and main concern, which type of primer seems best for you?**

- ► Hydrating
- ► Mattifying
- ► Pore-minimising
- ► Color-correcting

4. **Action plan:**

- ► Write down the type of primer you think will work best for you.
- ► Next time you apply makeup, follow the CTMP routine and observe how the foundation smoothly glides on your face and how the primer affects your overall look.
- ► Reflect on how your makeup looks after a few hours. Did it stay in place? Does your skin look smooth? What could be improved?

Primary Knowledge Quiz

1. What is the primary function of a makeup primer?
    - a) Adds colour to your makeup
    - b) Moisturises the skin
    - c) Creates a smooth base for makeup and prolongs wear
    - d) Removes makeup at the end of the day

    (Correct answer: c)

2. Which type of primer is best suited for oily skin?
    - a) Hydrating Primer
    - b) Mattifying Primer
    - c) Illuminating Primer
    - d) Pore-Minimising Primer

    (Correct answer: b)

3. If you notice your makeup looks patchy after a few hours, what might be the cause?
    - a) Too much foundation
    - b) Skipping primer
    - c) Not using enough powder
    - d) Using a matte lipstick

    (Correct answer: b)

4. True or False: Applying too much primer can make your makeup slide off.

    (Answer: True)

5. What is the key step you should complete before applying primer?

    a) Foundation

    b) Moisturising

    c) Setting Powder

    d) Lipstick

    (Correct answer: b)

6. If you have combination skin, what would be the best approach to primer application?

    a) Use a mattifying primer all over the face

    b) Skip primer altogether

    c) Apply a mattifying primer to the T-zone and a hydrating primer on the cheeks

    d) Use a colour-correcting primer only

    e) Use an all skin-type primer

    (Correct answers: c and e)

Bonus Activity: "Primer Experiment" Challenge

Try out different primers (or use your current one) and document your experience.

Instructions:

- For makeup applications, use a primer and observe how your makeup looks after a few hours.
- Does your makeup stay in place better than when you don't use a primer?
- Does your skin feel smoother, less shiny, or more hydrated?
- **Reflect:** Write down which primer worked best after these trials and why. This will help you personalise your makeup routine based on experience.

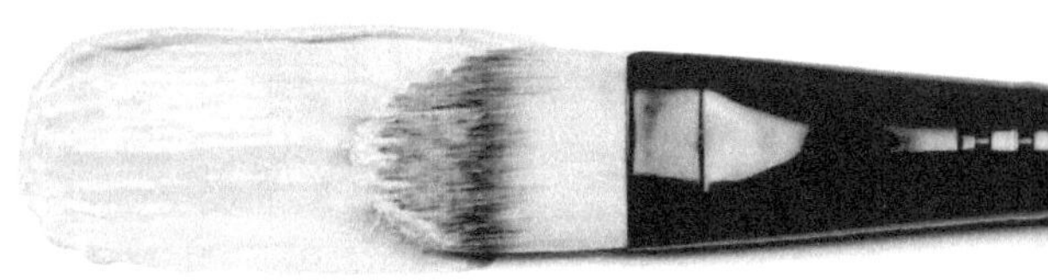

Chapter 4

Foundations – Find Your Perfect Match

It's called "foundation" because it sets the stage for your whole look. It creates a smooth base for all the following makeup—blush, bronzer, highlighter—helping everything blend effortlessly and last longer. Whether you want a natural glow or a more enhanced finish, foundation can help you achieve your desired look.

Levels of Coverage

Foundations come in different opacity levels, meaning how much of your natural skin will show through. Here's a quick guide:

- **Sheer Coverage**: Provides the lightest coverage. It's perfect for those who want their natural skin to shine through. If you love your freckles, this is for you.
- **Medium Coverage**: This product offers moderate coverage, which is great for evening skin tone while keeping a natural look. It covers some imperfections but still lets your skin's texture show.
- **Full Coverage**: Full coverage hides blemishes, dark spots, scars—anything you want to conceal—and gives an airbrushed finish. It's often the go-to for special events or photoshoots.

Foundation Finishes

Choosing the right finish is like picking the right outfit, depending on the occasion and your mood. Here are the main types of finishes:

- **Matte Finish**: This finish is ideal for those with oily skin or anyone wanting to keep shine under control. It gives a smooth, shine-free look.
- **Dewy Finish**: This finish is for you if you want a radiant, glowing complexion. It's perfect for dry or dull skin, giving it a hydrated, fresh appearance.

Types of Foundations

Foundations come in many forms, each suited for different skin types and preferences. Let's explore the options:

Liquid Foundation comes in water-based, oil-based, or silicone-based formulas with varying coverage (from sheer to full) and finishes (matte, satin, etc.). While it works well for most skin types, I personally find it tricky—it dries quickly, so you need to blend fast. Tip: Apply it in small sections and blend before moving to the next area.

- **Powder Foundation**: A lightweight, fine powder, often pressed, that typically provides a matte finish. It's ideal for oily or combination skin and can also be used to set liquid foundation. Growing up, compact powder was a staple in every woman's vanity. It was the easy, no-fuss solution for a hot, humid day, and I still reach for it when I need a quick matte fix.
- **Stick Foundation**: This creamy foundation in stick form is perfect for on-the-go touch-ups. It's my favourite travel buddy, offering medium coverage and working well for all skin types.
- **Cream Foundation**: Creamy, moisturising, and full coverage, cream foundation is my personal favourite. I love using cream foundations when I am at home and want to take my time getting ready. There's no rush with these; blend at your own pace and enjoy the process. This type of foundation feels luxurious on the skin.
- **Mousse Foundation**: Light and airy, mousse foundation blends easily and provides a matte finish. It's suitable for all skin types and offers light to

medium coverage. Personally, I find the finish a bit dull for my skin, so it's not my go-to.

- **BB Cream/CC Cream**: Lighter than traditional foundations, these creams are multitaskers—combining foundation, moisturiser, and SPF. BB creams are great for hydration and light coverage, while CC creams focus on colour correction. During wedding seasons, when I was still learning about makeup, these were my go-to. They were easy to apply and perfect for a quick, fresh-faced look.

- **Tinted Moisturiser**: For those who love the "no-makeup" look. Tinted moisturisers provide minimal coverage while offering hydration and a sheer finish. They're perfect for dry, normal, or oil skin. I used to rely on these when I wanted a hint of coverage.

There are also more options, like mineral and serum foundations, but I haven't tried them all. It's impossible to test every product on the market, but my advice is simple: if you're curious, do a patch test, get a sample size, and experiment.

Once I found what's right for me, I stopped further experiments. From the above list, cream foundations are my all-time favourite, and I use foundation sticks when I travel. Having a compact in my vanity is a habit—I cannot do my touch-ups without it.

Point of caution: Since the compact has a hint of colour, be mindful of where you apply touch-ups. Avoid doing touch-ups more than a couple of times, as it could lead to uneven patches of colour or make the makeup look cakey or overdone if not applied correctly.

Foundation Shopping Tips

I have learned over the years that if you don't know much about makeup, your shopping choices are often guided by the salesperson at the counter. They're there to help, but sometimes their goal is to sell you as much as possible. It's easy to walk out with more than you need. My advice? Go in with a plan, and don't let the sheer number of options overwhelm you.

Application Tips

There are different ways to apply foundation—brush, sponge, or fingers. I prefer a brush for cream and powder foundations, blending with a sponge for a smooth finish. For liquid and mousse foundations, I go straight to the blender. Early on, I would use a stippling brush and blend with a sponge, but now my routine is streamlined.

Finding the Right Shade

Choosing the right shade can be tricky, but here are some tips that can help:

- **Undertones**: Are you cool, warm, or neutral? If you have pink or red undertones, your veins appear bluish; you're likely cool-toned. If your skin has yellow or peach undertones, your veins appear green; you're warm-toned. Neutral is somewhere in between, where it's harder to tell—sometimes veins appear purple.

- **Test in Natural Light**: Always swatch the foundation on your jawline in natural light, not artificial lighting. It'll give you the most accurate match. Pick three shades and then see which blends seamlessly into your skin.

- **Watch for Oxidation**: Let the foundation sit on your skin for a few minutes to see if it darkens slightly after exposure to air. This helps you see how it truly blends with your face and neck.

- **Consider Seasonality**: Your skin colour might change slightly with the seasons—it might be darker in summer and lighter in winter. It's okay to have two different shades for different times of the year.

- **Mix Shades**: If you're between shades and having trouble finding a single shade, don't hesitate to mix two to find your perfect match. It's all about what works for you.

Each type of foundation has pros and cons, depending on the desired look and skin type. These tips should help you navigate the overwhelming world of foundations and find the one that enhances your natural complexion and boosts your confidence.

Reflective Activity: Your Makeup Journey

As you read about my makeup journey, grab a pencil and prepare to dive deep into your own! This activity empowers you to explore your unique makeup choices and discover what truly resonates with you. Take your time and answer the questions sincerely; your thoughtful responses will guide you towards finding your perfect makeup routine. I hope that by the end of this book, your answers will reveal realisations about the choices you make versus those you aspire to make, helping you rediscover the uniqueness within you.

1. **What skin type do you have?**

   (Oily, Dry, Combination, or Sensitive)

   My answer is: Dry to normal.

2. **Which finish do you prefer?**

   (Matte or Dewy)

   My answer is: Dewy.

3. **What level of coverage makes you feel most comfortable?**

   (Sheer, Medium, Full)

   My answer is: Before, I preferred sheer; now, I enjoy medium to full coverage.

4. **Describe a moment when you felt truly confident while wearing makeup. What foundation were you using?**

   I want to share a small incident that made a big impact. As mentioned in previous chapters, I rarely used makeup on my face. However, in 2017, I went shopping with a dear friend and came across BB and CC creams on the counters. Intrigued by the advertisements, we asked the salesgirl to show us how they looked on our skin. Following her advice, we purchased one according to our skin tones. After that, whenever we met, we complimented each other and laughed about the secret behind our newfound complementary looks. For a couple of years, I kept BB and CC creams in my vanity for rare occasions.

   Write your personal story here—it's a beautiful moment to reflect on!

5. **Reflect on your relationship with your skin. How has it evolved over the years?**

   I faced significant health issues from 2013 to 2022, which reflected on my skin, causing dryness, uneven tone, and blemishes. Little did I know, it was due to a lack of nutrition in my body. Once I found my teacher at the Natural Lifestyle Camp, everything changed. My skin improved, I felt better, and my energy levels increased.

   After learning about makeup, I realised my relationship with my skin has evolved. When I do my makeup, my skin looks better because I consciously take care of it before and after. My morning CTMB routine and night RCTMB routine have significantly improved the quality of my skin.

   My experiences have made me a strong believer in the importance of inner care as well as outer care.

6. **What do you hope to achieve with your makeup routine?**

   As a homemaker, I am least expected to be presentable while doing regular chores. However, my makeup routine brings me joy. When I am getting ready, it's me time, and it always makes me smile. I genuinely enjoy this— it's part of who I am.

Consider your aspirations; this could be about feeling beautiful, empowered, or simply expressing yourself!

Activities to Explore Your Makeup Preferences

Activity 1: Foundation Discovery

For the next month, try a different type of foundation each week. Keep a little diary of your experiences – how does each one feel? How does it look like as the day goes on? Reflect on how they enhance or alter your confidence!

Share your thoughts on how these foundations make you feel—does one bring out your inner glow more than others?

Activity 2: Foundation Inventory

Take a moment to assess your current foundation collection. What do you have, and what might you be missing? Create a checklist to categorise your products by:

- Type (Liquid, Powder, Cream, etc.)
- Finish (Matte, Satin)
- Usage (Daily, Special Occasions)

This is a chance to reflect on what you truly need versus what you might be holding onto out of habit.

Activity 3: Understanding Your Skin Tone

Let's get personal with your skin! Create a chart to categorise yourself based on:

- Skin Tone: Light, Medium, Deep
- Undertone: Cool, Warm, Neutral

Swatch foundations to find the perfect match for you! Remember, it's all about embracing your unique beauty and discovering what complements you.

"Remember, your makeup journey is personal, unique, and ever-evolving. Embrace it fully!"

Chapter 5

Colour Correctors for Blemish – Hiding and Concealers for Brightening

When used together, colour correctors and concealers can truly transform your complexion by addressing imperfections and enhancing your natural beauty. This chapter will explore how these powerful products can brighten and even out your skin.

Colour correctors can effectively address specific skin concerns. They work on the principle of colour theory. They help neutralise specific skin tones and create an even skin tone with the help of concealer, enhancing the overall appearance of the complexion.

It's important to pair a colour corrector with a concealer. Without concealer, using a colour corrector should be avoided as colour correctors neutralise unwanted tones, but they may leave behind a tint, which is why a concealer is essential to seamlessly blend everything with your natural skin tone.

My Story

I started learning about makeup products as part of my pageant training curriculum and bought a colour corrector because it was on the recommended list. However, I wasn't sure or confident about how to use it. I can imagine my readers thinking I must have Googled the information or followed some influencers, but those were different days. I wasn't a social media person then, and there was so much to learn that using a colour corrector didn't even make it onto my priority list.

During photoshoots, as makeup artists worked on the girls, I realised the magic that this duo—colour corrector and concealer—can create. When applied in the right amounts and blended perfectly into the skin, they create the illusion of flawless skin. Slowly, as I learned more, I began to love it just as much.

How Colour Correctors Work

Each colour corrector addresses a specific skin concern:

Colour correctors neutralise unwanted tones based on the colour wheel—opposite shades cancel each other out, like green neutralising red.

(Refer Colour Harmony illustration on page number 45)

- **Green**: Neutralises redness (e.g., from active acne, rosacea).
- **Peach/Orange**: Cancels dark circles under the eyes, especially on medium to deep skin tones.
- **Lavender/Purple**: Balances pale tones in the skin, helping to brighten and illuminate the complexion.
- **Red**: Helps neutralise very dark or black spots or moles.

Types of Colour Correctors

1. **Cream Colour Correctors**:
   - ▶ **Texture**: Rich and creamy, these are easy to blend and provide good coverage and extra moisture.
2. **Liquid Colour Correctors**:
   - ▶ **Texture**: Lightweight and often lighter on the skin and can be layered easily.

There are other options, like colour-correcting sticks.

Experiment and Practice: Finding the right shades and applying techniques may take time. Don't hesitate to experiment to see what works best for your unique skin. I like to stick to cream colour correctors, which give enough time to blend at one's pace.

Primary Colours:
Yellow
Red
Blue

Secondary Colours:
Orange
Purple
Green

COLOUR
CORRECTOR:
Use
complementary
colour as
Orange for Blue,
Purple for Yellow,
Green for Red

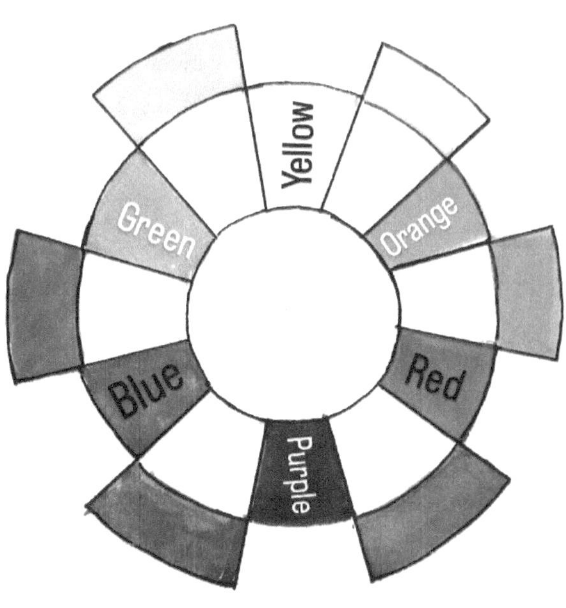

Pure Pigment: example:
Red, Blue etc

Hue + White

Hue + Grey

Hue + Black

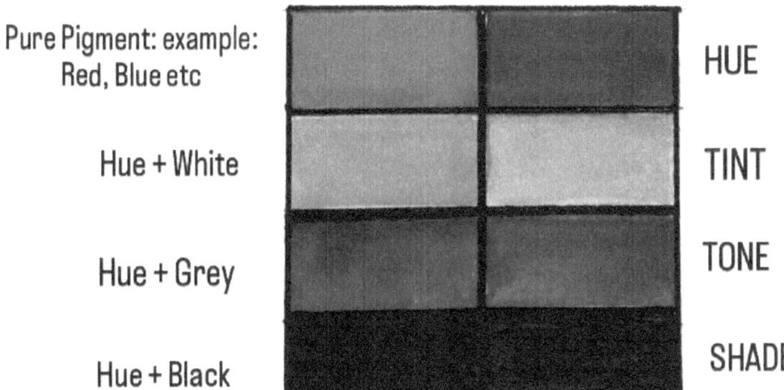

COLOUR HARMONY IN MAKEUP

Application tips for colour correctors:

1. **Start with Skincare**: Ensure your skin is well-prepped with the CTMP routine (Cleansing, Toning, Moisturising, Priming)

2. **Use Sparingly**: Less is more with colour correctors. Apply a small amount to the areas of concern (uneven skin colour) and blend well.

I use a brush to apply and then blend with a small blender.

Once you've neutralised unwanted tones with a colour corrector, the next step is using concealer to perfect the look and bring balance.

Now that we've covered colour correction, let's move on to the magic of concealers.

Concealer — for Brightening

Concealer is a makeup essential that can create a spotless complexion. It's your go-to product for brightening, hiding blemishes, and enhancing natural features.

Dark circles can make us look tired, and an uneven colour tone on the face makes us uncomfortable. When we apply a colour corrector to neutralise the uneven tones on the skin, our face looks unblemished.

Let's explore how to effectively use concealer to achieve that fresh-faced look.

Concealer is available in various formulations: liquid for light coverage (depending on consistency), cream for buildable coverage, and stick for convenience. It is important to choose the right shade to match your skin colour. For myself, I pick the one shade darker or the same shade as my skin tone.

Apply using your ring finger, a small brush, or a damp beauty sponge. Lightly dab the product onto the areas over the corrector and blend. This helps create a spotless surface and acts as a seamless transition between your foundation and concealer.

Highlighting and Contouring with Concealer

Once the unwanted tones are neutralised, concealers take the spotlight by enhancing your features and brightening your overall look. Concealer can be a powerful tool for highlighting and contouring.

Highlighting: Choose a concealer one or two shades lighter than your foundation. Apply it to the high points of your face, such as the under eyes, the centre of your forehead, the bridge of your nose, the philtrum, your chin, and a little bit on your temples. This brings attention to these areas and gives a radiant glow.

The key to successful highlighting and contouring is seamless blending.

Highlighting is one of my favourite steps because it can elevate the entire look.

(Refer to the illustration highlighting points on the face)

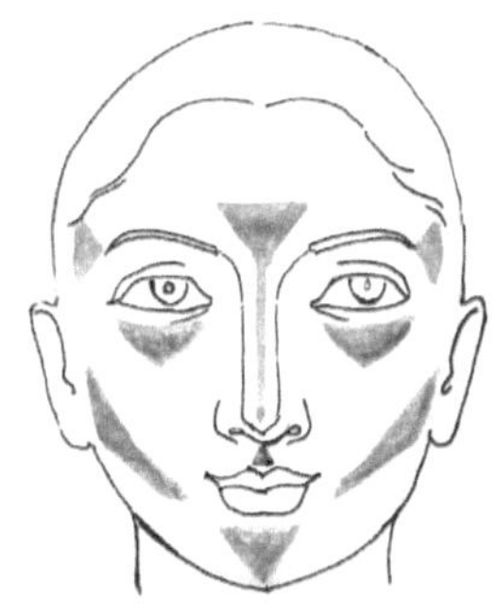

HIGHLIGHTING

Contouring: For contouring, select a concealer or foundation one or two shades darker than your foundation. Apply it to the hollows of your cheeks, along your jawline, on either side of your nose, and around the face to create an illusion. Blend well to create a shadow effect that sculpts your face.

To achieve a seamless look, use a damp beauty sponge or a brush to blend the edges of your highlighted and contoured areas. The goal is to create natural-looking shadows and highlights that enhance your facial structure.

(Refer illustration of contour points on the face)

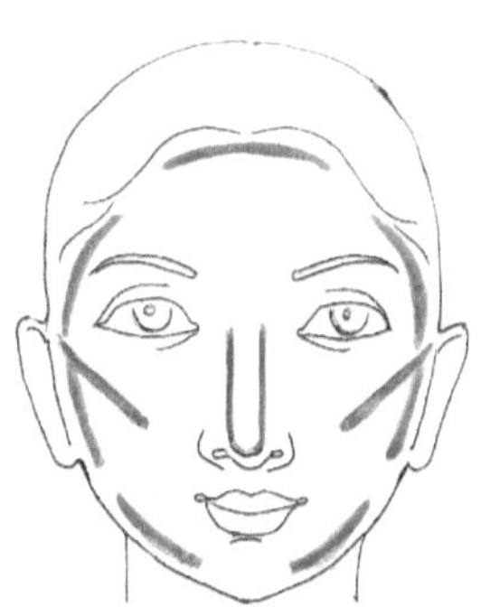

CONTOURING

Tips for Concealer Application

- **Less is More**: Start with a small amount of product and build coverage as needed. This prevents a cakey appearance.
- **Choose the Right medium**: Consider your skin type when selecting a concealer. Cream formulas work well for dry skin, while liquid formulas are great for oily skin.
- **Practice**: The more you practice applying concealer, the better you'll become at achieving a flawless finish. Don't hesitate to experiment with different techniques and products to find what works best for you.

Concealer stick in three different shades from light, medium to deep, is my constant travel buddy. I love it because of its versatility. When I don't want to use corrector for normal outings, I use concealer directly to cover the darker areas of my skin, especially under the eyes, around the lips, and the temple area. Then, a layer of foundation or lock it with compact or loose powder. When I am home, I prefer a cream formula. It can transform the look and help achieve a polished and radiant look. With the right techniques and products, you'll feel confident and empowered in your makeup journey.

Activity: Colour Correction and Concealer Quiz

Answer the following questions based on your knowledge of colour correctors and concealers. Reflect on your personal experiences and preferences as your answer.

1. **Colour Corrector Matching**:

   Which colour corrector would you use for the following concerns?

   a. Redness from acne

   b. Dark circles under the eyes

   c. Dull, pale skin

2. **True or False**:

   Colour correctors should be used alone without concealer.

   Personal reflection:

   Write down your favourite medium of colour corrector and concealer. What specific skin concerns do they help address? Describe how they improve your makeup routine.

Highlighting and Contouring Challenge

Using a concealer that is one or two shades lighter than your foundation, practice highlighting the following areas on your face (use a mirror for guidance):

- Under the eyes
- Bridge of the nose
- Chin
- After applying, take a moment to blend and observe the difference. How does this enhance your facial features?

Mastering colour correction and concealing take time, and the more you practice, the more confident you will become in your makeup journey.

Practice different techniques regularly and embrace experimentation with different products.

I encourage my readers to document their progress in a makeup journal to track which techniques work best for you.

Chapter 6

Setting Powder – Stay Flawless Throughout the Day

Setting powder is pivotal in ensuring your look stays fresh and flawless throughout the day.

It is a finely milled powder used to set makeup. It is made from absorbent material that helps control oil and ensures that makeup remains intact for hours.

It comes in an array of shades, each one with its magic, such as:

Translucent, coloured banana, illuminating setting powder, etc.

It should always match the colour of the foundation a person uses. One or two shades lighter work too.

Translucent powder is colourless, making it a no-brainer for setting makeup on all skin types without altering the colour.

Loose powder comes in various shades and can provide additional coverage.

Banana is a yellow-toned powder that works well for medium to deep skin tones.

Illuminating setting powder contains light-reflecting particles, giving skin a little sparkle and a radiant glow.

Use of Setting Powder

It keeps makeup in place for longer hours as it absorbs excess oil produced by sebaceous glands on oily skin and moisture effectively on a hot, humid day.

- *Keeps makeup intact:* Locks your foundation in place, preventing it from fading or smudging throughout the day.
- *Fewer touch-ups:* Once setting powder is well blended on your face, avoid touching your face for the longevity of the makeup without any touch-ups
- *Minimises shine:* For oily skin, this is an essential product that helps to achieve a matte finish.
- *Soften fine lines:* When used correctly, it minimises the appearance of fine lines by preventing concealer and foundation from settling into them, giving a smooth finish for makeup to look fresh throughout the day.

> Pro tip: I prefer to apply blush and eyeshadow after the setting powder absorbs the extra moisture on the skin for a more natural and lasting effect.

It acts as a barrier on your skin and prevents makeup from leaving a stain on the face. Any particles that drop on the under-eye area are easily dusted off without any need for touch-up.

When to Use Setting Powder

Every makeup artist has their own style, and they have streamlined it for themselves.

The way I like to use it is after applying a highlighter on the seven points (refer to the illustration on page no. 47). I have learned to use it on those points and let it sit for 10-15 minutes to allow the skin to absorb the layers of makeup, to give a touch-up to any visible fine lines. Blend it well on the highlighted points and all over the face with the help of a beauty blender. Then I move further to complete my makeup look with additional products like powder blush, bronzer, or powder highlighter.

Summers in the North of India, especially in Delhi NCR, are long and harsh. On no-makeup days, I prefer to carry setting powder with a small puff in my handbag to keep my face looking fresh on hot and humid days.

Incorporating setting powder into the makeup routine can significantly enhance the overall look.

> Tip: Ideally, avoid using liquid or cream products once the powder has been applied as this can disrupt the seamless finish.

Loose vs Pressed Powders: Which One to Choose?

Both **loose** and **pressed powders** differ in texture, application, and the results they deliver. They serve the purpose of setting makeup and giving a polished finish.

Let's explore the key differences between the two and help you decide which one best fits your needs.

1. **Texture and consistency**
   - ▶ **Loose Powder is lightweight and fine.**
     - It has a sheer coverage because of its texture and allows a natural finish.
     - Ideal for oily skin, it absorbs oil and controls shine.
   - ▶ **Pressed Powder:**
     - Pressed powders are solidified into a compact form, giving them a heavier, denser texture.
     - Pressed powder offers more coverage compared to loose powder, so it can be used for touch-ups or to build additional coverage.
     - Slightly Heavier on Skin: Because of its denser texture, pressed powder can feel a little heavier on the skin as compared to loose powder.

2. **Application and convenience**
   - ▶ **Loose Powder:**
     - Loose powder can be a bit messy due to its light, fine particles, therefore, it's best suited for at-home use or in situations where you have time to be precise.
     - You'll need a fluffy brush or a powder puff for application, and it's best to apply it sparingly for a soft, diffused finish. I have learned and practised to apply it with a beauty blender.
   - ▶ **Pressed Powder:**
     - Pressed powder is compact and easy to carry, making it ideal for touch-ups throughout the day. Most pressed powders come with an applicator sponge or puff, allowing for quick and convenient use when you're on the move.
     - Pressed powder because of its solid form; it's easier to control during application without spilling or wasting product.

- ▶ **Loose Powder:** Helps blur pores and imperfections.
  - ■ **Light to Sheer Coverage:** It provides sheer coverage, which is perfect for setting makeup without adding weight or extra colour.
  - ■ **Ideal for Baking:** Makeup artists often use loose powder for the "baking" technique, where the powder is applied heavily in certain areas (like under the eyes) on the top of the foundation. It is left on for 5-10 mins to set the make-up and absorb excess oil, then brushed away for a crease-free finish. Baking is the technique that saves makeup touch-ups and drips of powder sprinkled by mistake during eye makeup.

I absolutely love the sheer coverage it provides and the way it sets the makeup long-lasting without adding any weight or colour. I highly recommend this one for people who have oily skin or perspire more.

Personal insight

I gave the same suggestion to my daughter, who has an oily T-zone and perspires more in Chennai's (the southeast coast of India) climate. She absolutely loves it and kept my advice after she experienced its magic during her long hours of work.

- **Matte Finish:** Pressed powder gives a matte finish, but if not blended well, it can leave a more textured look.
- **Medium to Full Coverage:** Pressed powder provides more added coverage compared to loose powder. It can be used alone over moisturised skin or a light base or over makeup to set it.

Before I knew anything about loose powder, pressed powder was always part of my vanity. It gave the skin a polished look by providing a little coverage and a hint of colour. I always carried it in my handbag as I dabbed the puff to remove the sweat on my face.

Choices I make now:
- **For Loose vs. Pressed:** Pressed powder was my go-to for years. But once I discovered loose powder for baking, I preferred using it more, especially on those sweltering summer days!

- **For Cakey Look Prevention:** Learning to avoid that "extra white" look was a journey! I learned it hard to build thin layers, after many ghostly makeup mishaps.

Skin Types and Needs

- **Loose Powder:**
  - ▶ **Oily and Combination Skin:** Loose powder works best for oily or combination skin because of its ability to absorb excess oil and control shine without feeling heavy.
  - ▶ **Long-Lasting Wear:** It's great for those looking for long-lasting makeup since it helps lock in foundation and concealer.
- **Pressed Powder:**
  - ▶ **Dry to Normal Skin:** Pressed powder is better for dry to normal skin types, as it provides added coverage without drying the skin.

That's my skin type, and I absolutely loved it all my life as much as my mum loved it. I was always found picking it out from her vanity when I was younger.

- **Touch-Ups:** It's ideal for quick touch-ups throughout the day, making it easier to control shine or add a little coverage on the go.

I can vouch for the ease of using pressed powder.

Versatility and Uses

- **Loose Powder:**
  - ▶ **Setting Makeup:** Loose powder is primarily used to set foundation and concealer, giving a smooth, soft-focus finish that holds your makeup in place.
  - ▶ **Great for Baking:** Because of its fine texture, loose powder is excellent for setting the under-eye area and other parts of the face.
  - ▶ **Finishing Touch:** It's a great finishing powder after applying makeup to ensure a long-lasting, oil-free look.
- **Pressed Powder:**
  - ▶ **Dual-Purpose:** Pressed powder can be used as both a setting powder and a foundation for quick, light coverage. Works well for all skin types to blot facial perspiration.

> ► **Portable for Touch-Ups:** The compact nature of pressed powder makes it perfect for blotting oil for a refreshed look throughout the day.

My experience

While writing each chapter, my mind is replaying the moments of the beautiful journey I had. It was my 1st online session, along with other girls under training. During the makeup session, when the makeup artist asked us to apply setting powder generously, especially under the eye, a couple of us overdid it, and we looked like ghosts… hilarious… for a couple of months, I could not figure out how much was enough. I always ended up looking too white, like a ghost. But those were the days.

Our trainers were all judging us not for perfection but for the efforts we put in. I have pictures in that extra white look which I got through using generous amounts of loose powder. Not guilty or embarrassed of those faux pas; it is part of the learning process. We all learn through trial and error. And we continue to make mistakes until we figure out our own style.

Which One Should You Choose?
- **Choose Loose Powder if:**
  - ► You have oily or combination skin and need oil control.
  - ► You want a lightweight product to set your makeup for long-lasting wear.
  - ► You're looking for a natural, matte finish with sheer coverage.
  - ► You prefer using powder for baking or setting specific areas like the under-eye region.
- **Choose Pressed Powder if:**
  - ► You need something portable for touch-ups throughout the day.
  - ► You have normal or dry skin and want a product that adds some coverage without being too drying.
  - ► You want a quicker, less messy application.
  - ► You prefer a product that doubles as a foundation and setting powder.

Both loose and pressed powders have their unique benefits and uses. The choice depends on the skin type, makeup needs, and

personal preferences. You may even find that having both in your makeup collection allows for more flexibility depending on the occasion!

Have you ever felt unsettled in a cakey look?
Let's talk about how to avoid a cakey look.

The "cakey" look usually happens when the foundation or concealer settles into fine lines, clumps up, or sits on the skin unevenly. One can feel it after the foundation is done. It is visible after we use the setting powder and let it sit on the face; that's the time to check the status of the face if the fine lines are showing or camouflaged well. Here are some tips to avoid this and keep your makeup looking smooth and natural:

1. **Prep Your Skin Well**: Cleansing, toning, and Moisturising (CTMP) are essential steps for a smooth base. Exfoliating regularly also helps to remove dead skin cells, allowing makeup to adhere better. Choose a primer that suits your skin type, such as a hydrating primer for dry skin or a mattifying one for oily skin. (Sometimes excess facial hair acts as a barrier in achieving a smooth finish)

2. **Choose the Right Foundation**: Opt for a foundation with the right texture, finish, and shade for your skin type. For dry skin, a hydrating or dewy finish works best, while for oily skin, a matte or oil-free foundation is ideal. Make sure your shade matches to avoid visible layers.

3. **Use Thin Layers**: Applying multiple thin layers instead of one thick layer of foundation prevents the makeup from appearing heavy. Start with a light layer and build up only where you need extra coverage. Normally, one layer is sufficient; if needed, you can apply a second layer, but beyond that, it's your skill and preference. I usually try to stick to a single layer. For Bridal and full coverage many times more than one layer of foundation is applied. It also depends on the texture of the skin, makeup preference, and style.

4. **Blend:** Proper blending with a damp beauty blender can help remove excess product while pressing it softly with light hands into the skin for a seamless finish.

5. **Set with a Light Powder**: Using a translucent setting powder can lock your makeup in place and help avoid overdoing it. Focus on areas that tend to get oily (like the T-zone) and apply with a light hand. I blend it using a beauty blender.

6. **Use Setting Spray**: A setting spray adds a fresh finish to your makeup and helps it stay in place. It can also reduce the look of powder on the skin, keeping everything looking natural.

7. **Touch-Up as Needed**: If your makeup starts to look cakey later, lightly blend areas with a damp sponge.

8. **Practice is the key:** Practice enough to make sure that your handsets on doing all these steps flawlessly and quickly.

Initially, I started with 40-45 minutes until this step, and doing complete makeup looked like a herculean task. But now I can complete a look in 40-45 minutes.

A Quick recap:

- **Which powder is Right for You?**
  - ▶ Loose Powder: Sheer coverage, matte finish, ideal for oily skin
  - ▶ Pressed Powder: Buildable coverage, convenient for touch-ups, great for normal to dry skin
- **Tips for a Flawless, Non-Cakey Finish**
  - ▶ Prep skin, blend well, use light layers, and finish with a setting spray.

Let's reflect: Think about your daily makeup routine. Do you need long-lasting oil control or a quick touch-up?

- Jot down which setting powder (loose or pressed) suits your needs best based on your lifestyle.

Fun thought:

- ▶ Looking back, I can't help but laugh at my 'powder ghost' phase. Today, setting powder is my secret weapon for a fresh, lasting look, even in Delhi's heat! That's why I call setting powder makeup's best friend. There is a type for every vibe, and once you find your style, you'll feel makeup-ready for any occasion.

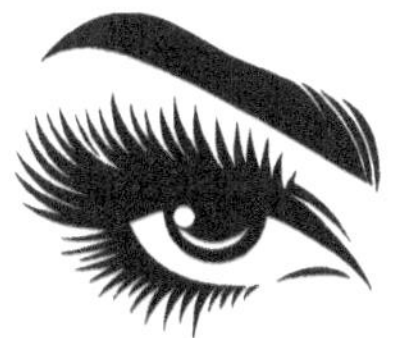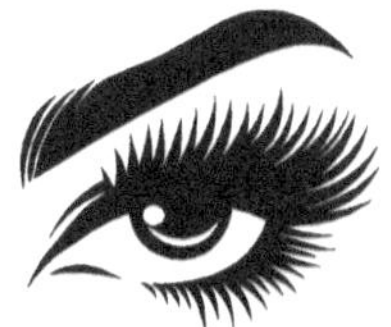

Chapter 7

Eye Makeup and Contact Lenses

Before adding depth and drama to the eyes, let's discuss contact lenses, which offer convenience and comfort for vision correction and cosmetic enhancement. If you wish to wear lenses, consider wearing them before applying makeup to avoid particles getting trapped under the lens.

For the national pageant, I had done my portfolio shoot without lenses. I was introduced to disposable contact lenses during my portfolio shoot for the International Pageant, which created a completely different look. I look at it as a unique element in how we present our eyes to the world.

Daily Disposable Lenses

Description:

Daily disposable lenses are intended for single-day wear. After a full day of use, they are discarded and replaced with a new pair the next day. Unlike reusable lenses, they don't require cleaning solutions or special care, making them convenient for occasional use.

Benefits:
- *Hygiene:* No risk of contamination since users start with a fresh pair each day.
- *Comfort:* disposable lenses are designed to provide comfort throughout the day.
- *Convenience:* easy to use, no maintenance, making them ideal for busy lifestyles.

Tips for Using Disposable Contact Lenses

- *Proper Handling:*
  - ▶ Always wash and dry your hands before handling contact lenses.
  - ▶ Avoid lotions or oils on your hands, as these can cause irritation.
- *Follow the Recommended Wear Schedule:*
  - ▶ For daily disposables, read the instructions and wear them only for the recommended duration (usually one day).
  - ▶ Do not sleep overnight with your lenses. Remove the lenses if you intend to sleep.
- *Eye Care Routine:*
  - ▶ Just as we do regular health checkups, keep in touch with eye care professionals to monitor eye health and hygiene if you regularly wear lenses for aesthetic purposes.
  - ▶ If there is discomfort with the lenses or any vision concerns, consult a professional.
- *Makeup Tips:*
  - ▶ Apply any makeup only after putting in lenses to avoid particles getting trapped under the lens.

Now that we've covered the basics of disposable lenses, let's talk about coloured lenses that can add versatility to the look.

Coloured Contact Lenses

These lenses are available in daily disposable options and can enhance or completely change your eye colour. With a wide range of colours, including black, brown, grey, blue, green, hazel, and turquoise, you can create a specific look for special occasions or costumes. Personally, I find hazel complements my warm skin tone beautifully. During my pageant journey, this is the colour I used most of the time for my photoshoots, and I absolutely love the look.

Application and Removal Techniques

- *Applying Lenses:*
  - ▶ Ensure your hands are clean and free of dust. Sit in a well-lit space for better visibility.

- *Removing Lenses:*
  - ▶ Wash your hands with soap. Ensure there is no dust or grime on your hands. Gently pinch the lens to remove it from the eye using your index finger and thumb.
  - ▶ It is advisable to consult an eye care professional for personal consultations for the care of lenses and the eyes.

Reflecting on my own journey, I recall my memorable firsts:

As a young woman, I loved experimenting with makeup and lenses. I remember when disposable lenses were new to the market around the year 2000, I bought every colour available. Those were reusable lenses, which required extra care for preservation. Back then, my vision was 6/6, and my spirits were high as a mother of young children. I practised wearing and removing them without hurting my eyes. Once, while going out for dinner, I wore blue lenses with a blue outfit it was not well received socially, though I felt confident and happy. I even had my hair streaked blond and burgundy. I was always fashion-forward, enjoying creative touches like studs or crystal rings on my long nails. My unconventional style wasn't always appreciated, but it brought me joy.

Now, 24 years later, I feel a thrill at the thought of wearing coloured lenses again. Although I had forgotten how to put them in quickly, I practised and regained the confidence to wear and remove them with ease. I personally like hazel and dark brown, and I think grey suits me too.

To me, fashion is pure fun, a happy place where creativity can shine every day. When my daughter went to college in her second year, I gifted her a pack of lenses with a range of colours, including cat's eye and purple. She enjoyed wearing them as much as I did and explored various streaks in her hair. As I write this book, her hair is streaked with blue and dark pink.

Safety and Hygiene Practices

- *Travelling:* When travelling, carry a couple of pair of lenses in case you would want to experiment on the go.
- *Adapting to New Lenses:* gradually increase the wear time until you become comfortable.

- *Emphasis on safety:* Since lenses directly impact eye health, ensure lenses are not expired and avoid sharing lenses with others.
- *Professional Guidance:* Be in contact with an eye care professional for advice, especially while exploring the new lens trends. Seek professional advice if it is your first time.

There are various types of lenses available in the market; I use coloured disposable ones. Pick the ones that suit your preferences. Wearing coloured lenses is an empowering choice—do what makes your soul happy. When our soul is happy, we look beautiful and feel confident.

Reflective questions:
- How do I feel when I wear lenses?
- Do I notice any changes in my confidence, mood, or style?
- What motivates me to choose certain lens colours?
- Do I pick colours based on trends, comfort, occasions, or mood?
- How well do I maintain a clean and hygienic routine when handling my lenses?
- Are there any steps I could improve to keep my eyes healthy?
- Have I noticed any issues or discomfort when wearing lenses?
- How have I managed this, and could I do anything to prevent it in the future?
- What have I learned from my past experiences with lenses, and how has that shaped my current choices?
- Do I adjust my eye makeup when wearing certain lens colours or styles?
- How comfortable am I with the process of applying and removing lenses?
- Do I have any personal tips or routines that make this process smoother?
- Who am I going to contact during an emergency? Do I have any details of an eye care professional handy in my contact list?

Eyeshadow – Adding Depth and Drama

Makeup Pairing

Eye makeup should always complement the colour of the lenses. For example, using lighter, more neutral eyeshadows can create a natural look with brown or black lenses, while vibrant colours make a statement with coloured lenses.

Choosing Shades for Your Eye Colour

- **Brown Eyes:** Brown eyes are incredibly versatile, allowing for both warm and cool tones. Rich shades like copper, bronze, and burgundy bring warmth and enhance the natural depth of brown eyes, while soft pinks and purples add a delicate richness.

  The reason I am suggesting these colours is that browns are a safe bet whether you use them during the day or in the evening. Pinks and purples can enhance elegance or add a little drama depending on the shades and tones you pick and their placement.

- **Blue and Green Eyes:** Blue eyes pop with warm tones like copper and coral, making them stand out with brightness. Cooler shades can work as well but may require blending for a soft finish. For green eyes, shades that match their warmth or create contrast—like plum, rust, or gold—bring out their natural charm. Check the colour wheel online or in-store to find inspiration for complementary colours to get ideas and remember that experimenting and practising will help you find what works best.

  Colour choice is entirely personal, and there's no wrong choice – it's about expressing your personality in a way that feels authentic to you.

- **Hazel Eyes:** Hazel eyes suit a variety of shades, making them ideal for creating dynamic looks. Browns with a touch of shimmer can add elegance, while a hint of highlighter near

  The tear ducts or shimmer on the lids can make hazel eyes sparkle beautifully.

Blending Techniques for Day and Night Looks

Day Look:

1. **Base Colour**: Start with a neutral shade matching your skin tone across the lid to create an even canvas.

2. **Highlight**: Apply a light shade to the inner corners of the eyes and beneath the brow bone to brighten the eyes and create an awake and refreshed look.

3. **Define the Crease**: Use a mid-tone shade in the crease. For a natural effect, pick a shade slightly darker than your skin tone and blend softly with a fluffy brush. My go-to is always shades of brown, and I adjust the shade based on the colour of my outfit, occasion, and mood.

4. **Blend, Blend, Blend**: To achieve a polished look, blend any harsh lines using circular motions.

Don't worry if you don't achieve perfection at first. Remember, even pros refine their techniques over time!

> **Tip**: After finishing your eyeshadow, a setting spray can help lock in the look and prevent fading.

Night Look:

1. **Intense Base**: For a bolder look, start with a darker shade on the lid, like deep brown, navy, or black.

2. **Deepen the Crease**: Apply an even darker shade to the crease and outer corners, focusing intensity on the outer corner and blending well.

3. **Shimmer for Glam**: Tap a shimmer or glitter shade onto the centre of the lid to catch the light for a glamorous effect. Sometimes, you can use your fingertip to apply for a smooth finish.

4. **Liner and Lashes**: Complete the look with eyeliner and mascara, adding definition and drama.

> **Tip**: For special occasions, try experimenting with coloured liners or false lashes to elevate your look even more.

My Experience

I prefer not to write too much detail about day and night looks because makeup is a practical skill that is best learned hands-on. I suggest finding the right mentor who can guide you through self-application, as it's a technique that truly benefits from a trained eye for a flawless finish. While makeup enthusiasts can certainly watch lessons from influencers on social media, there's nothing quite like personalised guidance.

There are various types of eye makeup looks—smoky eyes for a party, natural makeup for everyday wear, halo eyes, cut creases, and many more. My favourite is the cut crease, where I love to play with shades of brown for a natural effect. I have found that applying makeup on the eyes often takes the most time; blending the right colours to achieve the desired result is key.

In my own journey, I experimented with different eye makeup techniques through online videos, but it was only through proper training that I truly understood the craft. This training helped me create my own style and gain the confidence I needed.

Let me share a bit of my story with you to provide some clarity. My very first lesson was online, involving a theoretical foundation and a list of items to prepare for our next session. I asked my daughter to help me order the products, and while she suggested buying smaller quantities, I stuck to the list to avoid any embarrassment since many of my co-contestants were half my age or younger. Meeting online meant we didn't know each other well until we gathered for our training sessions. Honestly, I was overwhelmed by the sheer number of products on my table—and let's just say my "powder ghost" experience was hilarious!

> *Pro Tip:* Start small with essentials and gradually expand your collection as you grow comfortable.

Over time, I sought lessons from various professionals, but I often left feeling uncertain about my skills. I needed someone with an organised and structured training format who could genuinely guide me. That's when I discovered Bhumika Bahl, a passionate teacher of this beautiful art. She nurtures her students and even nourishes them with good thoughts and good food, unlike any other trainers I have come across so far. I witnessed firsthand how her students leave her academy with newfound confidence and financial independence.

I went there seeking knowledge, and I found exactly what I wanted. This knowledge, combined with my experience as a pageant queen, gave me the confidence to write this book.

Learning makeup is like learning to dance, paint, or play music—first, we build our foundation so we can confidently grow in the right direction. Makeup is a skill, a creative outlet, and even a hobby for many young girls who love to look beautiful and enjoy a little touch-up here and there. I encourage every makeup enthusiast to seek guidance from a mentor who inspires you. This way, you're not only prepared for life's occasions but also able to hold your head high if anyone questions your skills. You can confidently say, '*Trust me, I know what I'm doing.*' To me, that is empowerment—owning your craft without a second thought.

Finding a good mentor makes all the difference in makeup, as in any art. If you're feeling uncertain, remember we all start somewhere. There's so much beauty in the journey of learning and growing.

Embrace every step of your learning journey—explore different colours, celebrate each look you create, and step forward with confidence. Like I found my style in cut creases and warm browns, I hope you find what makes you feel beautiful and authentic.

For eyes, one can learn more by watching less and practising more. Reading helps the least in eye makeup.

Reflective Questions:
- What shades did you feel most confident wearing?
- Did you find any unexpected favourites?
- How did blending different shades change your look?

Eyeshadow enhances one's natural beauty. Remember, makeup is an art form that should be enjoyed and personalised. There are no fixed rules. Find what resonates with your soul and own it.

Eyebrow Products – Framing Your Face

When the eyes are expressive, words become unnecessary. With the right makeup, the eyes make a powerful statement, and the eyebrows provide a perfect frame. Whether soft or bold, they help define your personality.

This realisation came to me during one of my makeup training sessions. The artist defined the brow on one side of her face, leaving the other side untouched. I could immediately see how the right shape and shading in a brow can transform the entire look of the face, adding subtle sharpness. After this, I noticed with other artists as well that eyebrows need attention for a well-defined look. Before this, I wasn't a fan of doing my eyebrows beyond simply combing them to keep them neat. But now I have learned how impactful well-defined brows can be.

Different Tools: Pencils, Powders, Gels and Brushes

Once the eyeshadow is applied, it's time to give the finishing touch by enhancing the eyebrows for a well-defined look. Each eyebrow tool works differently to achieve the desired result:

- **Pencils:** Ideal to fill in sparse areas and define the brow shape. Some pencils have brushes attached on the other end to give eyebrows a neat look with precise strokes.
- **Powders:** Create a soft, natural finish by adding fullness without harsh lines, perfect for a subtle look.
- **Gels:** Keep brow hairs in place, clear gels provide a simple hold. While they don't add volume, they keep brows in place for longer hours. I prefer using it with a spoolie attached that provides a simple hold. Rarely do I fill my eyebrows with tints.
- **Wax:** Eyebrow wax keeps your hair in place throughout the day without making them stiff. Apply it with a spoolie for a clean brow shape. I prefer using clear wax to maintain my brow shape. To add tints, I fill them with powder or pencil, depending on my mood and what I can quickly grab from my kit.

These tools can be mixed or used alone to achieve anything from natural to bold brows, depending on the look you want.

Eyebrow Brushes

Eyebrow brushes are essential for shaping, blending, and refining brows. Let's talk about different types of eyebrow brushes and their uses:

- **Spoolie Brush:** This mascara-like wand is perfect for brushing through your brows to blend products, soften lines, and shape the hair. It's great for prepping brows before applying the product and blending afterwards for a natural look.

- **Angled Brush:** With its precise, angled tip, this brush is ideal for applying powder to fill in sparse areas and define the brow shape. It's also helpful for creating sharp lines or enhancing the arch.

- **Dual-Ended Brow Brush:** Often combining an angled brush on one end and a spoolie on the other, this tool allows you to apply, shape, and blend products for a polished look. This brush is my favourite pick as it reduces the need for multiple tools, making it convenient for quick application.

- All these tools work well in defining the brows. Ultimately, it's a personal choice to pick what you are most comfortable using.

  (Refer to the illustration on Page no. 109 in Chapter 14)

How to Start and Which Colours to Pick

It's advisable that eyebrows should not be darker than your hair colour; avoid using black. Dark brown or light grey makes a good choice. To shape the brow, always start from the middle and go towards the end first, then move from the front to the centre at the bottom of the brow. Use a similar approach on the top of the brow, ensuring you give the desired shape to the arch.

To fill the brow, always start from the centre and move outward in the direction of the brow hair. With a gentle touch, fill the gaps, and then come to the front, making upward strokes to ensure each strand is separate and not sticking together. Slowly, with soft strokes, move outward.

Once it's done, finish with concealer or foundation along the brow line using a flat, thin brush for a polished look.

There is no secret formula or theory on how it should be done; this is a practical skill to develop. Again, you can look into tutorials on social media to find techniques that resonate with your style.

Eyeliner: Defining the Eye

Eyeliner is a powerful tool in makeup that can enhance the eyes, define their shape, and create a range of stunning looks. Whether you prefer a bold wing or a subtle line, understanding the different types of eyeliners and their application techniques is essential for achieving your desired effect.

In everyday life, if we observe girls, they like to wear eyeliner to define the shape of their eyes and mood. That flick tells a lot about a person, their personality, and mood, doesn't it?

Types of Eyeliner

1. **Liquid eyeliner:**
   - **Description:** Liquid eyeliner comes in a small bottle with a brush or felt tip applicator to control the amount of product dispensed. It has a thin, fluid consistency, to allow smooth lines on the eyes.
   - **Finish:** It typically dries to a long-lasting, matte, or shimmery finish.
   - **Best For:** Creating sharp, defined lines and dramatic looks, such as winged eyeliner.

2. **Pencil eyeliner:**
   - **Description:** Pencil eyeliner is available in both traditional wooden and retractable formats. It comes in a creamy texture that makes it easy to glide over the lid.
   - **Finish:** It can provide a matte or shimmery finish.
   - **Best for:** A more natural look, easy blending, and quick application. It is ideal for beginners due to its user-friendly nature. Sometimes, it comes with a smudge brush on the other end, which makes it more user-friendly.

3. **Gel eyeliner:**
   - **Description:** Gel eyeliner comes in a small pot and is applied with a brush. It has a smooth smudge-proof creamy texture that glides on easily.
   - **Finish:** It offers a semi-matte finish and lasts longer than liquid eyeliner.
   - **Best For:** Creating a soft, blended look or a more defined line, making it versatile for both day and night looks. It can be used to create smoky looks.

Eyeliner looks:

There are various ways to play with eyeliners, allowing you to create different moods and styles.

Beginners can stick to basics and experiment as their skill develops.

- *Natural eyeliner—or, as I learned to call it, tight liner—is a thin line made from the beginning to the end of the upper lash line. It's perfect for everyday wear, quick, and* subtle.

- *Winged liner:* Use a flick that goes past the upper lash line towards the temple. Depends on how far and how dramatic you would like to be.

- *Peacock liner*: I call it a peacock liner. To me, it looks like that when a thin line comes from the upper lash line and makes a fine beak-like point before merging with the lower lash line and a flick that goes past the upper lash line towards the temple. This adds a little drama, good for bold evening looks.

Understanding Eye Shapes

Understanding the shape of your eyes is the key to highlighting their natural beauty. Each eye shape has unique characteristics that can be highlighted with the right makeup techniques. Below is a guide to various eye shapes, tips, and my take on how to enhance them.

1. **Hooded eyes:**
   - ▶ **Characteristics:** The eyelid is partially or fully covered by a fold of skin, making the lid appear smaller.
   - ▶ **Enhancement Tips:** Use lighter shades on the lid and darker shades in the crease to create depth. Winged eyeliner can help elongate the appearance of the eyes.

   To me, these eyes look most beautiful in my favourite cut crease eyeshadow.

2. **Monolid Eyes:**
   - ▶ **Characteristics:** Lack of a defined crease gives a smooth, flat eyelid appearance.
   - ▶ **Enhancement Tips:** Apply light and shimmering shades on the lid to create dimension. Define the lash line with eyeliner and emphasise lashes with mascara for an open look. I have not worked on such eyes but what I see in pictures is kohl-rimmed dark colour gives definition to the eye while light colours make eyes look bigger.

3. **Small Eyes:**
   - **Characteristics:** Smaller than average, these eyes can often appear more delicate.
   - **Enhancement Tips:** Use lighter, shimmering shades on the eyelids to open up the eyes. Apply eyeliner on the inner rim to make them appear larger and focus on mascara to emphasise the lashes.
   - Light-coloured kajal makes eyes look bigger.

4. **Big Eyes:**
   - **Characteristics:** Larger than average, attracts all the attention.
   - **Enhancement Tips:** Use darker eyeliner on the outer edges to create a definition. You can also experiment with bold eyeshadow colours according to the occasion.
   - Kohl: Applying black or dark kohl along the waterline makes the eyes look beautiful and more attractive.

5. **Droopy Eyes:**
   - **Characteristics:** The outer corners may sag slightly, giving a more relaxed appearance.
   - **Enhancement Tips:** Brightening the inner corner with a highlighter is a good idea.

6. **Close-Set Eyes:**
   - **Characteristics:** The distance between the eyes is less than one eye's width.
   - **Enhancement Tips:** Using lighter shades on the inner corners and Winged eyeliner looks good and can help create the illusion of more space.

7. **Wide-Set Eyes:**
   - **Characteristics:** The distance between the eyes is greater than one eye's width.
   - **Enhancement Tips:** Apply darker eyeliner on the inner corners. Peacock eyeliner complements these eyes. Focus on connecting the inner and outer corners with eyeshadow to create the illusion of less space.

8. **Upturned Eyes:**
   - ▶ **Characteristics:** The outer corners are higher than the inner corners.
   - ▶ **Enhancement Tips:** Emphasise the outer corners with darker shades to accentuate the upward shape. Winged eyeliner enhances the shape of the eye.

9. **Downturned Eyes:**
   - ▶ **Characteristics:** The outer corners are lower than the inner corners.
   - ▶ **Enhancement Tips:** A tight liner can give definition to the eye.

Enhancing Your Eye Shape

Once you observe, understand, and accept the shape of your eyes, it becomes easier to enhance their beauty by using the right shades and liners. My favourite part of eye makeup is working on the crease line, blending perfectly, and creating a beautiful gradation. I especially enjoy enhancing the look by adding a touch of shimmer on the lids, which draws attention to the overall appearance. Experiment with different techniques and colours to find what works best for you. Remember, *there are no rules, makeup is all about expression and creativity,* so have fun while enhancing your unique features!

Kohl

Kohl, known as *kajal* in Hindi, has been used in India for centuries, passed down from one generation to another. It is a cultural staple from newborns to the elderly. Kohl in India is more than cosmetic. It is an embodiment of tradition.

Aesthetic and Beauty Enhancement

- In India, Kohl enhances the natural beauty of large and expressive eyes. Kohl-filled eyes are often seen as a mark of beauty in Indian culture.
- Traditional Indian bridal makeup relies heavily on kohl to create a bold, dramatic look for the eyes. For married women, kohl signifies beauty; it has a cultural significance as part of the *solah shringar* (the 16 traditional beauty adornments).

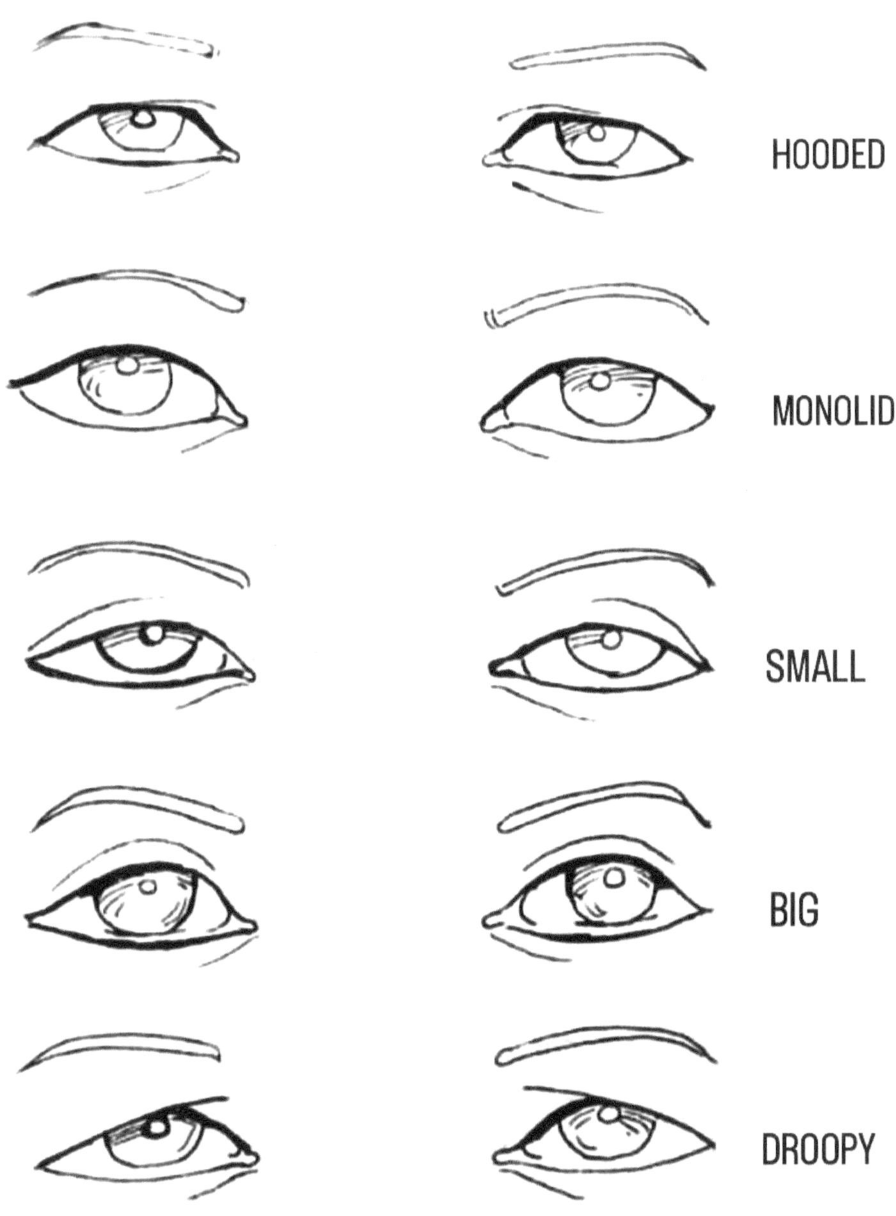

DIVERSE EYE SHAPES

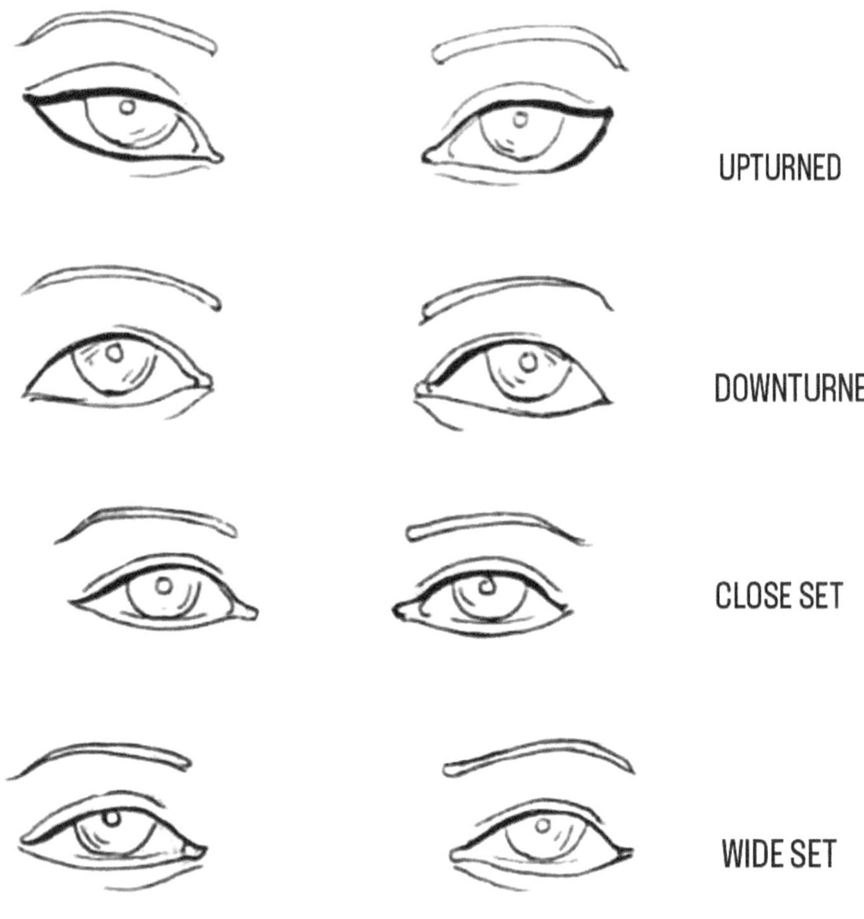

DIVERSE EYE SHAPES

Medicinal Properties and Eye Health

Traditionally, homemade kohl was created from natural ingredients believed to have cooling and medicinal properties. Many believe that applying kohl can protect the eyes from infections, soothe irritation, and even improve eye health.

Embracing Kohl in Your Routine

Kohl remains one of the most popular products, suitable for everything from casual to glamorous looks that make the eye look captivating. Whether you like a soft smudged line or a bold statement look, kohl can bring out the natural beauty of your eyes. Its timeless appeal and ease of use make it an ideal choice for any makeup lover's collection.

Key Characteristics of Kohl

- **Soft Texture:** Kohl is typically softer than many other eyeliners, making it easy to smudge for a smoky look or to apply precisely for defined lines.
- **Intensity:** The deep pigment in kohl provides a bold colour, ideal for dramatic or traditional looks.
- **Versatile Application:** Kohl can be applied on the waterline, lash line, or even blended onto the eyelid for a quick smoky effect. I use it to blend onto the eyelid for a smoky effect and top it with a layer of darker powder.

How to Use Kohl

1. **For a classic look:**
   - ▶ Gently apply kohl along your upper and lower waterlines. This gives a traditional look that defines the eyes.
2. **Smudged or smoky effect:**
   - ▶ Apply a thick line of kohl along the upper lash line and blend it outward using a brush for a smoky look.
3. **Winged Kohl look:**
   - ▶ With a kohl pencil, draw a wing at the outer corner of your eye, then use a round brush to blend and soften it gently. This technique merges the boldness of kohl with the sophistication of a winged finish.

4. **Inner corner highlight:**
   ► Balance the intensity of the kohl with a touch of highlighter in the inner corner to make the eyes appear bigger and more elegant.

Tips for Wearing Kohl

- **Set It with Powder**: If you have oily skin or find that kohl smudges easily, set it with a matching eyeshadow to help prevent smudging throughout the day.
- **Avoid Overdoing It on Small Eyes**: Since kohl can be intense, keep it minimal or use nude colour on small eyes. Try to pair it with a lighter tint on the lids.
- **Experiment with Colours**: Kohl is available in many colours, like brown, nude, blue, green, and more. Each adds its own unique flair to the eyes.

Like many girls, I was fond of kohl-rimmed eyes. Even though I don't have oily skin, my kohl would always smudge after a short time. Despite this, my love for kohl never faded. Over time, however, I developed concerns about dry eyes and was advised by my doctor to avoid putting kajal, which led me to switch to gel liners.

Initially, this transition was challenging; I was so accustomed to seeing myself with kohled eyes that without them, I felt incomplete. But as I stopped using kajal and embraced eyeliner instead, I gradually found peace with my new look. With time and experience, I have learned to appreciate my eyes in a different way, feeling confident and beautiful without the kajal.

False Eyelashes

While Kohl enhances eyes naturally, for a more dramatic transformation, false eyelashes are a great option. They instantly add shape to the eyes and bring length and volume to natural lashes, creating a glamorous look. They are perfect for those with shorter lashes or sparse lash lines, filling in gaps to make lashes appear fuller. Synthetic lashes are most commonly used, especially for special events.

Application Steps:

1. Apply a thin layer of lash glue along the band, letting it dry for 15-20 seconds until it is ready to stick and stay.

2. Place the lash at the centre of your upper lash line, then gently press it down on the outer corner and finally the inner corner.

3. Once set, finish the look with eyeliner, checking for any gaps in the inner and outer corners for a seamless finish.

Removing False Lashes:

Gently peel them off, starting from the outer corner and moving towards the inner corner, and store them carefully for reuse.

Mascara

Mascara is a user-friendly essential for defining lashes by giving them a darker appearance and added volume. I find my lashes tend to be less curled, but with the use of mascara, they achieve a perfectly lifted look—something I truly love about this product, making it suitable for both every day and glamorous styles, especially when paired with false lashes.

There are different types of mascaras: for lengthening, volumising, curling, and waterproof formulas, which are ideal for hot, humid days or water shoots.

Application Tips:

1. **Upper Lashes**: Start at the base of your upper lashes. Look straight ahead and rest your lash on the spoolie, wiggling the wand as you move upward to coat each lash evenly.

   ► For the right side, look left, rest the right side of the lashes on the spoolie, and wiggle the wand upward.

   ► For the left side, look right, rest the left side of the lashes on the spoolie, and wiggle upward.

2. **Lower Lashes**: Look up and place the spoolie on your lower lashes, slowly moving downward.

3. Use the tip of the spoolie for hard-to-reach areas, like the inner and outer corners.

4. If you would like to apply 2 or 3 coats, then allow each coat to dry before applying the next to avoid clumping.

Removal:

Use a gentle eye makeup remover, especially for waterproof formulas. Soak a cotton pad, press it gently against your lashes, and swipe downwards to remove.

Now that we've explored the key concept of eye makeup, it's time to move from learning to experiencing. Let us take a step-by-step approach to create a simple eye makeup look. This exercise will help us understand the sequence of products we have read about so far.

1. Preparing the eyes: Start with a pea-sized amount of primer for even application on your eyelids to create a smooth base and ensure long-lasting wear.

2. Use a colour corrector if there is any uneven skin tone on the eyelids and crease area (as per the intensity of your skin tone, use peach or orange colour).

3. Apply concealer to create an even skin tone, and blend well using a brush, blender, or finger (I prefer to work with a small blender on the eyes).
    Pick a shade that matches your skin tone.

4. Foundation to create the base (use blender for an even finish)
    Normally, this step is relevant when we are doing a full makeup look; we can skip it for now.

5. Dab translucent powder and let it sit for ten minutes and let the skin absorb the moisture. This can help absorb excess oil, especially for those with oily eyelids. Otherwise, we will find cream settled in lines after we finish doing the eye makeup.
    Remove extra powder from the surface and blend well using a blender, you can now spritz setting spray too.
    Note: These are the normal steps we follow when we are doing a complete makeup.

6. For quick eye makeup, we can skip these steps and use a cream eye base of the colour you want for your eyeshadow. Then follow the following steps.

I recommend using a brush or blender for application, although there are artists who use fingers as well for application. Personally, I like to use a damp small beauty blender.

> *Tip:* Remember to always lock the creams or liquid base with powder for a long-lasting look.

7. Pick a neutral shade from the eye palette (powder) that matches the colour of the skin and add a seamless base to the eye with a round fluffy brush.
8. Take a darker shade of brown and apply it on the crease line. Blend well on the crease line using a round brush and making circular motions.
9. Take a lighter shade, apply it on the eyelid, and blend well. There should not be a visible harsh line between the colour of the crease line and the colour of the eyelid.
10. Use a nude colour or a lighter colour just under the arch of the brow and blend well with the crease line. There should be a gradation effect, with no harsh lines visible. It gives the eyebrow an enhanced and lifted look.

Note: Draw an imaginary line from the inner eye corner to the beginning of the brow and the outer eye corner to the end of the brow. Your colour blending should stay within this boundary. This helps maintain symmetry and balance.

1. Once the eyes are done, work on shaping the brows and filling them as told in the chapter. Remember to use brow wax or brow gel whatever is available in your vanity for a neat finish.
2. Kajal (optional) can be applied on the water line. Or can be used as a hidden liner for a subtler effect.
3. Put on the lashes (optional).
4. Apply eye liner. Ensure both the eyes look even and there is no gap between the liner and the lash line (skin is not visible). Start with the thin line and gradually increase the thickness to achieve the desired look.
5. Finally, use mascara to finish the look. Remember to rest your lashes on the spoolie and wiggle it while making an upward movement. You might want to consider using two coats for more volume and a lasting finish.

Final touches:

Make a note of mistakes.

1. Applying too much product or a lack of blending will leave harsh lines.
2. Use a Q-tip with makeup remover for any errors and try to fix them
3. Check out the pictures on Google and pick your favourite style of liner you would like to practise.

My Story

I have a progressive eye condition, which makes it essential for me to rely on glasses. I do not wear vision correction lenses, as they make me more prone to falling when climbing or descending steps or uneven surfaces. This limitation makes it difficult for me to do any eye makeup with finer details. It took me some time to overcome this challenge, but now I have streamlined my style.

I do not use kajal because of dry eyes, and due to my vision, I find it challenging to achieve a fine finish in the inner corner of the eye. However, if someone can do it for me, I love getting a normal simple liner done. It remains my favourite. My eyelids have unique folds, and the presence of crow's feet doesn't complement winged liner as much.

Instead, during my training while learning different ways of playing with eyeshadows, I found my love in the cut crease look, often without liner or kajal. On rare occasions, I do like to apply nude kajal. I sometimes enjoy a soft smudged under-eye effect. This journey has taught me that makeup is not just about following trends; it is an ongoing journey. The more you practice, the better you become, the more you want to explore. Makeup has given me the confidence to discover my preferences.

This book is not just for reading and learning. It is crafted with the intention of active learning through activities. It is meant to be experienced. I invite you to engage in the learning process as an active participant fully.

Don't just read the book; experience the book.

Activity: Vanity Exploration

Before moving on to the next chapter, take a moment to explore your vanity. This chapter has covered many elements used for eye makeup, so it's the perfect time to check what you have.

1. **Inventory Check:** Look through your products and make a list of everything you own for eye makeup.

2. **Experimentation:** Try using all the products in your collection. This activity will help you assess the utility of each item and identify any gaps in what you have versus what you may need.

3. **Documentation:** As you experiment, take notes on what you like and dislike about each product. This will assist you in making informed decisions in the future about what to keep or replace.

4. **Reflection:** After trying out your products, reflect on your findings. Ask yourself:

   ▶ What did I enjoy using the most?

   ▶ What products do I feel are missing from my collection?

   ▶ Based on these reflections, consider if you need to upgrade your vanity to enhance your eye makeup skills further.

   ▶ Check the expiry date. The print is often too small and can easily be overlooked.

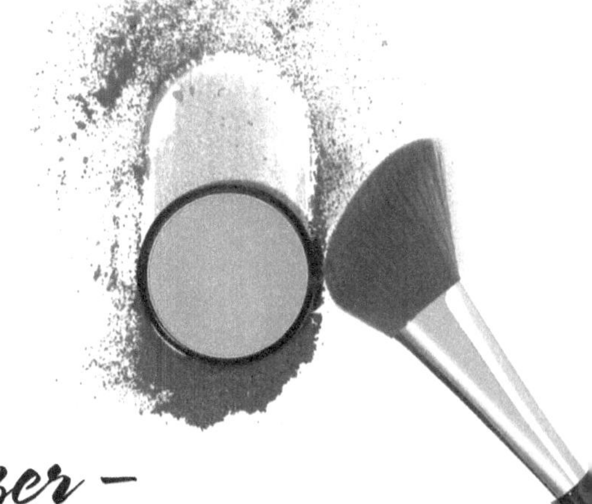

Chapter 8

Contour & Bronzer – Sculpting Like a Pro

In this chapter, we'll explore the art of contouring and bronzing to enhance your face's unique structure.

Contouring creates an illusion of depth and definition, while bronzer adds warmth and glow. When these two products are used together with perfection, they work magically to highlight your features subtly.

Defining Your Face Shape with Contour

Before contouring, it's important to understand your face shape. Start by taking a photo of yourself without any makeup for reference. This will help you assess your features and guide you towards balanced contouring to achieve the desired look. First, understand your face shape before picking the product.

Face Shapes and contouring tips.

1. **Oval Face** – Light contouring along the forehead and jawline to enhance natural balance. A touch of contour below the cheekbones adds a gentle definition.

2. **Round Face** – Contouring along the sides of your face, below the cheekbones and jawline, creates a sculpted look.

3. **Square Face** – To soften the angular feature Contouring at the edges of the forehead and along the jawline gives a softer illusion. A slight shadow under the cheekbones adds dimension.

4. **Heart Face** – Contour along the sides of your forehead to balance the upper face. Light touches along the chin are best avoided, as they can add sharpness.

5. **Oblong Face** – A horizontal application of contour at the top of your forehead, below the cheekbones and under the chin create a subtle definition and the illusion of an oval face.

Contour vs Bronzer: When and How to Use Both

- **Contour**: Used to define and sculpt, the contour is typically two to three shades deeper than your foundation. Apply contour in targeted areas like the hollows of the cheeks, along the jawline, sides of the nose, forehead, and temples. Remember, blending is essential for a natural, enhanced look that defines your bone structure.

- **Bronzer**: Pick a bronzer shade that complements your skin tone, giving the skin a radiant, sun-kissed soft glow. Ideally, apply bronzer to the areas where the contour is applied. Start by applying a small amount and build up gradually to avoid an overly bronzed look.

Pro Tips for Flawless Application

Now that we have understood how to apply contour and bronzer, let's talk about tools and techniques to ensure a seamless finish.

- **Choose the Right Tools**: For bronzer, use a fluffy brush to create a soft, diffused effect. A fan brush can also provide a luxurious, airbrushed finish.
  My experience: When I started, I used to load up my fluffy brush with too much product, which resulted in a patchy glow. Trust me, the initial struggle with finding the right amount of product is real. But with practice, you get the hang of it and improve over time.

- **Blend Well**: Avoid harsh lines by blending your contour and bronzer thoroughly for a seamless finish.

- **Less is More**: Start with a small amount and build up to your desired glow gradually.

- **Set with Powder**: A translucent powder is the secret to a long-lasting finish. Lightly dust it over your liquid contour and liquid bronzer for a polished look.

This finishing step is one of my favourites because it brings a soft, natural radiance without feeling overdone. Try it yourself and see how it enhances your glow!

When experimenting, pay attention to the finish. Some bronzers can leave shimmery patches, so choose one that gives a natural glow without being too obvious.

Activity Time

- Note your face shape and try enhancing areas that bring out your natural beauty.
- For makeup enthusiasts, this can be a fun weekend activity at your favourite store! Experiment with different pigments and find your glow.

When used together, contour and bronzer work like magic to bring out your inner goddess, subtly enhancing your features in beautiful, natural ways.

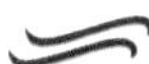

Chapter 9

Blush – The Rosy Flush

A pop of colour on the cheeks makes the face look lively and attractive, adding a youthful touch. In this chapter, we'll discuss how to choose and apply the right blush for your skin tone, creating the perfect finishing touch.

Types of Blushes

Blush comes in a variety of colours and formulations. Remember to start with a small amount and build up slowly, blending upwards as it's easier to add more colour than to remove excess from the face.

Powder Blush

Description: Powder blush is one of the most common types, ideal for oily and combination skin, offering a matte finish.

- Application: Use a round, fluffy brush to apply it. Dab softly from the cheeks to the temples while smiling, ensuring the colour is placed correctly. Then, blend gently for a soft, diffused look.

Cream Blush

Description: Cream blushes are often available in palettes or tubes with a variety of shades. They're ideal for dry and normal skin.

Finish: Dewy, providing a healthy, radiant flush.

- Application: Cream blush is easy to blend to create a dewy finish. Blend upward using your fingers or, preferably, a beauty blender.

Liquid Blush
- Description: Liquid blushes have a thin consistency and often come with a dropper. They are highly pigmented; a few drops are enough for a dewy finish. They blend smoothly into the skin.
- **Application:** Liquid blush can be used for intense colour. Start with a single drop and then build by blending with your finger or a sponge. This medium is my recent favourite.

> *Tip:* If you choose to use liquid or cream blush, always remember to lightly set it with a matching powder blush for a longer-lasting finish.

Now that you know your skin tone and the available formulations, choose from a wide range of colours, from peaches and corals to pinks and deeper pinks. Blush creates the illusion of lifted, fuller cheeks with a pop of colour. Learn to apply it in the right places for the desired effect.

Once you understand the different types of blushes, the next step is choosing the right shade for your skin tone.

Choosing the Right Shade of Blush for Your Skin Tone
- **Light Skin**: Light pinks, peaches, or corals look beautiful on light skin, enhancing the cheeks with a diffused look.
- **Medium Skin**: Go for warm tones of peach and pink to complement the natural warmth.
- **Tan/Deep Skin**: Rich, pigmented colours like deeper pinks or warm reds add brightness to the complexion.

Placing Your Blush

Blush placement can make a big difference in how your overall look comes together. Think of blush as a way to enhance your face. It's like adding a little life to your face.

- **Classic Cheek Apples**: Smile gently and apply blush to the apples of your cheeks. This is the most natural look that brings a gentle warmth to the face. This is how I have used my blush all my life.
- **Lifted Look**: For a modern look, apply blush slightly higher on the cheekbones, closer to the temples. Blending it upwards with a blender or brush gives the face a lifted appearance. This is my latest favourite way to apply blush for a polished look.
  When I first tried the lifted blush look, I wasn't sure how it would turn out. But after blending it well and stepping back, I noticed how it made my face look fresh and polished.
- **W Blush**: Adding a soft colour to the bridge of the nose, going all the way from the cheeks to the temples. I love this look for its outdoor, sun-kissed vibe.

Some people like to put a hint of colour on the tip of the nose and chin. I like it too sometimes. There are more ways to apply blush. Experiment and pick your favourite through testing and trial.

Always remember that in makeup, less is more. Blend well to achieve a natural look. Use a brush, blender, or your fingers for your preferred finish. Choose a colour that complements your overall makeup look.

How I have Used Blush All My Life: I would pick a lipstick shade and dab a bit of the same tint on my cheeks, blending it with my fingers. I picked up this simple hack from my mother, and it served me well over the years. It's always been my go-to for a quick, one-minute look. Have you ever tried using your favourite lipstick as a blush? Give it a go and see how it transforms your look with minimal effort.

Blush for Every Age

Blush is my secret to instant radiance. It not only brightens my face but also uplifts my mood, whether I am in a rush or taking my time to perfect my makeup.

Here's how it can work wonders across different stages of life:

- Over 50: It adds warmth to mature skin and a youthful glow without settling into fine lines.

- Ages 36-50: This will make you look refreshed throughout the day, reducing the appearance of tiredness.
- Ages 20-35: A quick 5-minute hack to amp up the look while juggling work-life balance.
- Teenagers: Perfect for a fresh natural look with or without minimal makeup. It was my personal favourite for school or casual outings.

Experiment with different shades and techniques, and find what works best for you. Whether you prefer a bold pop of colour or a soft, diffused glow, blush is a versatile product that can enhance your natural beauty at any age.

Reflect and Practice

While you experiment with different colours and placements, take notes on what feels most authentic to you.
- How does each shade enhance your cheeks and make you feel?
- Do you prefer a natural, softer look or a bolder look with a pop of colour?

I hope you're keeping a journal to track your findings, reflections, and realisations.

Embrace this journey to discover your personal style with me. By the end of this book, you'll be amazed at the knowledge you've gained to create your own curated makeup collection, choosing products that truly suit you.

Have fun with colours as we continue this makeup journey together!

Chapter 10

Lips – Defining Your Pout

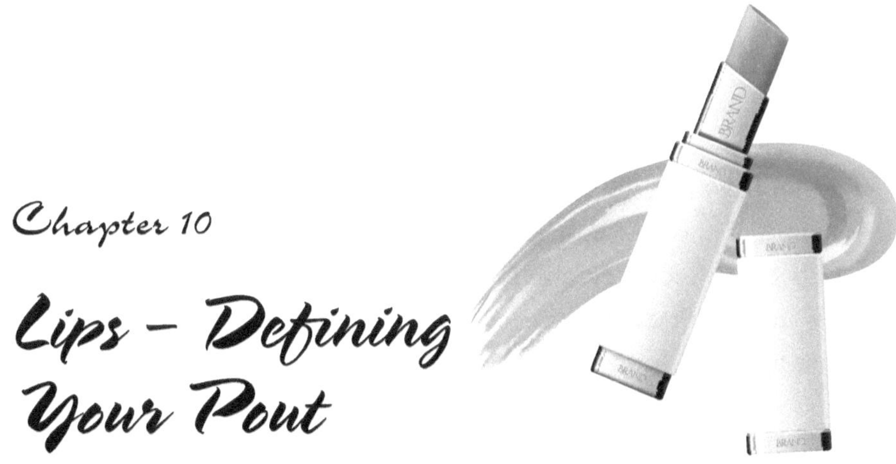

Lip liner is both a tool and a product that defines the perfect shape of the lips, enhancing the longevity of lip colour by creating a solid base. In this chapter, we'll explore using lip liner as a base, the lipstick application techniques, and how to finish with a glossy touch for a polished look.

Lip Liner: The Foundation of a Defined Pout

Lip liner not only provides a seamless outline to the lips but also serves as a long-lasting base for lipstick. Its creamy texture makes it easy to apply and gives lips a matte, defined look. Here are some tips for using lip liner effectively:

- **Outline Your Lips:** Draw along your natural lip line, or for a fuller-looking look, slightly over-line by tracing just outside your natural lip line. This technique adds volume while keeping the look subtle.
- **Fill for a Solid Base:** After outlining, fill in your lips with the liner to help prevent your lipstick from fading or bleeding throughout the day.

Lipstick: Colour and Precision

Using a lip brush can elevate your lipstick application.

1. **Use a Lip Brush:** Start with a lip brush instead of applying directly from the lipstick tube. This technique creates a thin, even layer that reduces the chances of smudging throughout the day.

2. **Dab Away Excess cream**: Lightly press a small round brush against your lips after the first coat to remove any excess product. This extra step gives your lips a polished, elegant finish, making the colour last longer.

Experimenting with different techniques can show you just how transformative lip liner can be. It enhances your lip shape, helps colour last longer, and creates a polished yet natural look. This section encourages you to look beyond simply picking a colour and applying it from a tube; it's about exploring textures, finishes, and methods to achieve your desired look.

Matte vs Glossy Finishes: Choosing Your Lip Look

Lipsticks come in a wide range of colours and finishes, each creating unique effects.

- **Matte Lipsticks**: matte lipsticks offer a long-lasting, smooth, elegant look without any shine.

- **Glossy Lipsticks**: Glossy lipsticks add shine, giving lips a radiant, dewy effect that's perfect for a fresh, vibrant look.

Choosing between these finishes is all about finding the style that best suits your mood or occasion.

Finding Your Perfect Shade

Selecting a favourite shade is a fun process that allows you to express your personality. Here are some helpful tips:

- **Consider Your Skin Tone**: For warm tones, try corals, peaches, and warm reds. Cool tones pair well with reds or soft pinks.

- **Test and Try**: Testing shades in-store or at home helps you see how they look in different lighting and how they wear over time.

- **Choose for Occasions**: Lighter nudes and pinks are great for everyday wear, while bold red makes a statement for evening events.

Personally, I love soft pinks and nudes for casual get-togethers. My go-to is a sheer pink shade that gives a natural, polished look. I like to reapply a thin coat every few hours to keep my lips looking fresh.

Choices I like to make:

Over the years, my love for makeup never faded, and I still enjoy wearing vibrant colours. I feel alive, surrounded by colours! I remember in 2019, my daughter and I went to Bhutan, and on every trip together, we try to do something fun and different. This time, we planned to go bold and vibrant in our choice of lipstick colours. We wore unique shades: green, turquoise, yellow, dark purple, and many more. This activity brought so much joy that we started our day with excitement, laughter, and giggles, confidently sporting our quirky colours. We had so much fun watching people turn their heads and compliment us.

Have you tried something quirky, experimented, and played around in a way that brought a smile to your face and the people around you?

Lip Gloss:

Lip gloss is a holy grail for adding shine to the lips—there's truly nothing else like it! Not only does it create a luminous look, but it also provides hydration and gives the illusion of plumper lips. It's my absolute favourite for the sparkle it adds.

Adding Dimension

Creating dimension with lip gloss is all about placement and layering:

- **Highlight the Centre**: After applying cream lipstick, dab a small amount of gloss in the centre of your lower and upper lips. This trick enhances shine and gives the illusion of fuller lips, while also intensifying the colour.
- **Hydrating Formulas:** Hydrating glosses leave lips looking soft and supple, though they may require reapplication throughout the day to maintain their shine.

Types of Gloss

Lip glosses come in tinted and non-tinted varieties, both of which work beautifully to enhance the lips. Tinted glosses add a subtle pop of colour, while non-tinted glosses provide a natural, glossy glow. Both can create either a subtle sheen or a full, glamorous shine.

Choose the right gloss and apply it in a way that can give your lips a unique, beautiful finish every time. Personally, I love wearing gloss over my lipstick whenever I step out; it completes my look and adds an extra touch of shine!

Chapter 11

Highlighter – Glow Like a Diva

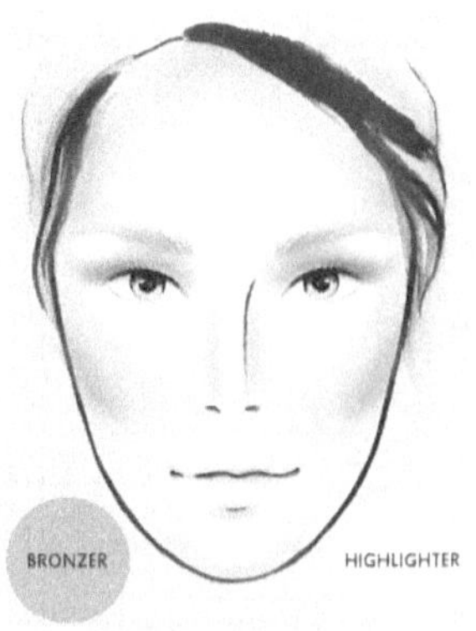

Highlighter is a magical product that brings subtle radiance to the face. It can transform your look, making you glow like a diva.

Liquid vs. Powder Highlighters

Whether you're aiming for a subtle glow or a bold shimmer, there are several highlighter options to choose from.

- **Liquid and Cream Highlighters**: These blend well and give a natural, dewy finish. They work well for normal to dry skin types. Such highlighters add hydration and radiance for a soft glow. I love them for their seamless finish.

- **Powder Highlighters**: Powder formulas are buildable, allowing you to achieve a more intense glow. They work well on oily or combination skin types and are ideal for a long-lasting glow.

> **Tip**: Choose your glow according to the occasion—soft and subtle for daytime, or a more striking glow for evening events. Always lock the liquid or highlighter with a light dusting of powder for a long-lasting look.

Placing the Highlighter

Here's a guide to achieving a naturally radiant look:

- **Cheekbones**: Apply on cheekbones for a lifted, sculpted effect.
- **Bridge of the Nose**: A subtle highlight along the nose bridge adds definition.
- **Tip of the Nose**: A subtle highlight on the tip of the nose with a fingertip for a subtle glow that brings attention to the centre of the face.
- **Brow Bone**: Highlighting under the brow arch gives a lifted appearance to the eyes.
- **Cupid's Bow**: Adding a touch on the cupid's bow creates a fuller, plumper look to the lips.
- **Inner Corners of the Eyes**: This brightens your eyes, making you look more awake.
- **Chin and Collar Bones**: A touch on the chin or collarbones adds dimension and a soft, natural glow if they're visible in your outfit.

> **Tip**: Start with a light touch. Tap off excess product from the brush, apply with soft strokes, and build gradually as needed. Avoid applying too much highlighter at once. It's easier to add more than to tone it down, ensuring a more natural, radiant glow.

Techniques for a Flawless Glow

- **Using a Sponge for Liquid and Cream**: Use beauty blenders to apply liquid or cream highlighters for a flawless, even finish. This technique gives a lustrous, luxurious, seamless glow. (For a quick touch-up, gently blending with your fingertips can also work well, especially for cream highlighters). I personally prefer using a damp beauty blender.
- **Using Brushes for Powders**: A dense fan brush works well with powders, blending them more smoothly than a sparse brush
- **Blending**: No matter which type you use, blend the edges carefully to avoid harsh lines and create a naturally radiant glow.

Choosing Your Perfect Shade

Highlighters come in a variety of shades that can enhance different skin tones:

- **Light Skin**: Champagne or silver tones add a natural, radiant glow.
- **Medium Skin**: Golden tones bring warmth and richness to your complexion.
- **Deep Skin**: Bronze or gold highlighters create a stunning glow that complements deeper skin tones.

Personal Reflection

Experimenting with highlighter can add elegance to your look and elevate your style. Highlighters have become my new favourite way to play with makeup. I love the glow it gives, enhancing both my look and my confidence!

I hope reading this book makes you feel like learning something from someone who has personally experienced the joy of makeup.

Activity: Discovering Your Glow Style

Describe your ideal glow style in a few words. Are you drawn to soft glam, or do you prefer a bold, shimmery statement look?

Chapter 12

Setting Spray – The Secret to an All-Day Fresh Look

As we are coming closer to the completion of this book, this is the last chapter on products to buy while creating your vanity.

No matter the occasion or the weather, setting spray is essential for maintaining your desired look.

Why Setting Spray is Essential for Long-Wear

Creating a flawless makeup look takes time and effort. After perfecting our makeup, we want it to last without fading or sliding off. Setting spray helps to lock in your makeup, ensuring it stays throughout the day. My makeup has stayed over 10-12 hours during my pageant weeks, and that is when I realised why professionals swear by this product after creating a piece of art. This realisation solidified its place as an absolute essential in my vanity.

Here are some key benefits of using setting spray:

- *Longevity:* Helps prevent smudging and fading. It works like a protective barrier over your makeup.
- *Hydration:* Some formulations help keep your skin looking fresh, dewy, and hydrated, especially in a dry environment.
- *Finish:* You can achieve a matte finish or a more radiant look.

How to Apply Setting Spray for Different Skin Types

Apply the setting spray correctly in order to retain its effectiveness. Here's how to do it based on your skin type:

- **For Oily Skin**: Use a matte setting spray to control oil and reduce shine.
- **For Dry Skin**: Opt for a hydrating setting spray.
- **For Combination Skin**: An all-skin type setting spray is ideal.
- **Application**: Spray 8-10 inches away from your face to allow the mist to spread and sit evenly across your skin.

Tips for Maximum Effectiveness

- **Layering**: A light mist after applying foundation can create a smooth canvas for further applications.
- **Dampen the Sponge**: Spritz setting spray on a sponge to blend foundation, concealer, or setting powder for a seamless finish.
- **Reapply throughout the Day**: A quick spritz of setting spray every couple of hours can refresh your look.

Personal Reflection

Setting spray is my secret weapon for achieving a fresh makeup look all day long. I truly appreciate its ease of use and purpose. I often find myself grateful to the formulator for their thoughtfulness and vision in creating a product that helps me stay vibrant and presentable on busy days and special occasions.

Be it the hot summers of Delhi NCR or the harsh, humid heat of Chennai; this has become my go-to essential before stepping out of the house.

Setting Spray vs Finishing Spray

They may sound or look similar, but they have a purpose of their own.

Let's find out the difference between the two:

Setting spray

1. It is designed to help makeup last longer.
2. It can be used between the layers of makeup to prevent sliding off the previous layer while building the layers.
3. It prevents makeup from smudging or fading.

4.   Perfect to wear in hot or humid weather for a long-lasting look.

5.   Use the formulation keeping in mind your skin type.

6.   It works well as a final touch in case one runs out of finishing spray and is available in ranges that can provide a matte, dewy, or shimmery look.

Finishing spray

This is the final touch on your face, giving the makeup a polished look.

1.   It gives a luminous, dewy, or matte finish as per the preference. I personally like the one that gives a dewy finish.

2.   It makes your face feel tighter compared to the setting spray. That's one of the reasons for avoiding its use between the layers.

Setting spray is used in between the layers to enhance the longevity of the makeup while finishing spray is the final touch to provide a matte, dewy, or shimmery look.

Activity

To find your favourite setting spray, try testers in stores one at a time, at least once a week, and note how each enhances your makeup look.

A Note to the Men

We all deal with changing weather and often rely on a handkerchief or towel to wipe our faces or freshen up. But have you considered spritzing some setting spray before heading out?

- **Situation 1:** Start with your favourite moisturiser or lotion, just as you usually do. Then, finish with a spritz of setting spray for that extra touch of freshness.

- **Situation 2:** Apply your moisturiser or lotion as usual, then set it with a loose translucent setting powder. Allow it to sit for about 10 minutes to absorb any excess oil or moisture on the surface. Afterwards, gently remove any excess powder and finish with a setting spray.

Try this out on a relaxed day at home and see how you feel. If it keeps your face looking fresh, it's a great way to elevate your everyday look, whether at the office or a party!

If this piques your interest, I encourage you to read Chapter 2, **CTM - Your Skincare Essentials.**

And guys, do you think this skincare routine is just for women?

Cleansing, toning, and moisturising can make a huge difference for your skin too. A simple routine can keep your face looking fresh, clear, and well-groomed, whether you're prepping for a date or just want to feel confident in your everyday look.

Here's a bonus idea:

If you are still not ready to try it for yourself, why not gift this book to the women in your life: your girlfriend, wife, daughter, or mother? It could help them make informed makeup choices and avoid unnecessary purchases, saving them (and you) from falling prey to persuasive sales tactics at the beauty counter. Trust me, they'll thank you later, and you will be grateful for this idea.

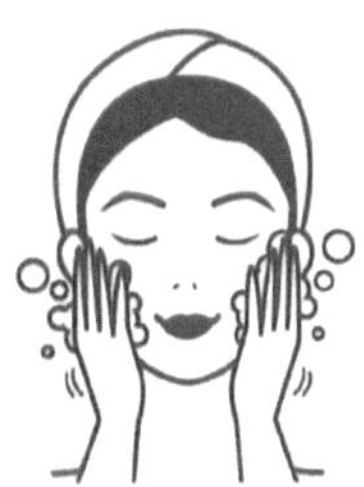

Chapter 13

Makeup Remover – The Final Essential Step

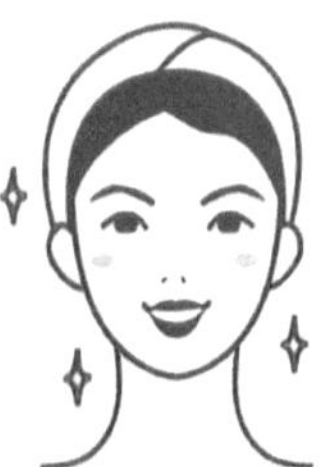

When we talk about makeup products, makeup remover is one product that often gets the least attention. However, it is one of the most crucial steps in a skincare routine.

The Importance of Proper Cleansing

Using the right makeup remover ensures that your skin remains healthy, and it can breathe once all the layers of makeup are removed. Choosing the right product to remove makeup maintains your skin's natural glow and prepares your skin for the future by removing debris that can clog pores.

How to Properly Cleanse Without Damaging Your Skin

1. **Be Gentle**: Avoid harsh scrubbing to prevent irritation on the skin.
2. **Use Cotton**: To prevent friction, use cotton or soft cloth or makeup remover wipes.
3. **Double Cleansing**: Start with an oil-based remover to break down makeup, then follow with a gentle cleanser to ensure every trace is gone.

Different Types of Makeup Removers for Various Skin Types

1. **For Oily Skin**:
   - ▶ Foaming cleansers help remove makeup while controlling excess oil

2. **For Dry Skin**:
   - ▶ **Cream-Based Removers**: Cream-based or lightweight oils dissolve makeup without stripping moisture.

3. **For Sensitive Skin**:
   - ▶ Look for fragrance-free removers designed specifically for sensitive skin types.

4. **For Combination Skin**:
   - ▶ Cleansing milk can effectively remove makeup while balancing the needs of both oily and dry areas.

Personal Reflection

Cleansing milk can effectively remove makeup while balancing the needs of both oily and dry areas. I feel it is really important how your skin feels day after day as you embark on your makeup journey. As you build your vanity kit, include a good makeup remover. A proper cleansing routine helps you enjoy the makeup journey without compromising your skin's health.

Remember not to let the excitement of applying makeup overshadow the importance of removing it at the end of the day. Taking charge of your skincare routine to maintain healthy skin is crucial. Makeup removal is an essential, yet often underappreciated step in the beauty routine.

Activity

To find the right makeup remover for your skin, try different products and observe how your skin reacts—look out for irritation, rashes, or breakouts. Make a note of what works for you and what to avoid.

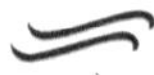

Chapter 14

Makeup Tools – The Trusted Allies

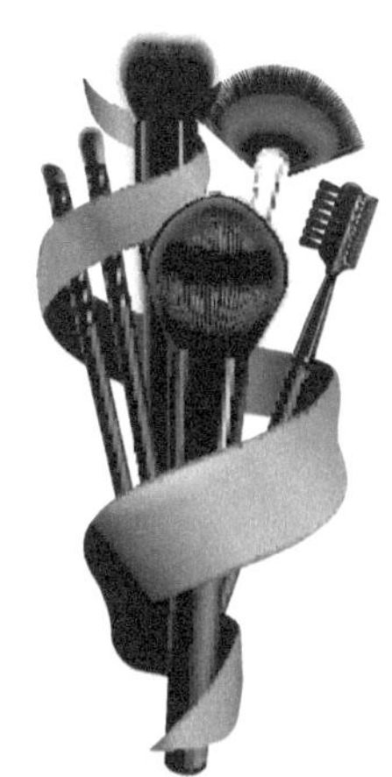

When discussing makeup products, it's common to overlook the tools required to apply them effectively. It's not entirely our fault; after all, using tools correctly requires training. With the right training, we gain knowledge that empowers us to make informed choices—whether in makeup or any other field. Without the right knowledge, we tend to rely on popular methods used by those around us, which might not always be the most effective.

Here is a list of essential tools for makeup:

1. Palette Knife and Mixing Tray

I hadn't considered a mixing tray as essential until I learned its correct use at Bhumika Bahl's academy. Using a mixing tray is one of the most hygienic ways to handle makeup products, as it avoids direct contact with hands.

For example:

- **Moisturiser**: Like many, I used to pump it into my hands and rub it in between my palms before applying it to my face resulting in half of it being absorbed by my palms. But now, I have learned the right way of application. I understand that proper hydration is critical for achieving a flawless makeup finish.

> **Pro Tip**: Shake your moisturiser before dispensing it onto the mixing tray. For optimal hydration, pump a generous amount, use a flat brush to emulsify it on the tray, and then apply it evenly on your face using a brush or fingertips.

Similarly, the mixing tray can be used to apply oils, primers, and foundations (whether cream or liquid).

Customised Makeup with the Mixing Tray

The tray also enables you to mix and create customised shades, whether it's for foundation, contour, blush, or cream lipstick. This level of customisation helps you achieve a perfectly matched shade for your skin tone or the desired look.

Using the Palette Knife

A palette knife is another essential tool for hygienic application. It allows you to keep your product free from contamination as you scoop products out of containers without repeatedly dipping your fingers.

Cleaning the Tools

After each use, wipe the mixing tray and palette knife with a wet wipe to keep them clean and ready for the next time.

2. Tweezers and Eyelash Tools

- **Tweezers**: Essential for shaping eyebrows and helpful when applying individual false lashes, especially for makeup artists working on clients. However, for personal use, many find that using hands is sufficient, especially for simpler lash applications.
- **Eyelash Curler**: Used to curl the lashes before mascara, creating a lifted, eye-opening effect.

> *Personal Tip*: While many use an eyelash curler, I achieve my desired effect by focusing on technique with mascara. I apply upward strokes firmly from the lash roots to the tips, which gives my lashes a natural lift without needing a curler.

3. Beauty Blenders

Beauty Blender/Sponge: This tool is ideal for applying and blending foundation, concealer, and cream products. I learned to use it to seamlessly blend setting powder for a smooth finish.

- **Choose the Right Size**: Use smaller sponges for precise areas like under the eyes and around the nose and larger blenders for broader areas of the face for efficient blending.

> Tip: Always use a damp beauty blender, making sure to squeeze out any excess water. If it's too wet, it may lift the product off your skin instead of blending it.

Cleaning the Beauty Blender

1. **Soak**: Place the blender in a mixture of baby shampoo and warm water. Let it soak for about 10 minutes to loosen product buildup.
2. **Rinse and Squeeze**: Rinse with clean water, squeezing out the colour and excess product.
3. **Repeat**: Soak it in fresh water for another 10 minutes, then rinse again. Repeat the process as needed until the sponge is clean.

Regular cleaning keeps your beauty blender hygienic and extends its lifespan, ensuring it's always ready for your next makeup application.

> Tip: When squeezing the blender during cleaning, be mindful that long nails don't dig into the sponge, as this can cause damage. If it gets cut or is damaged, it's time to replace it.

Brushes

A makeup brush in the hands of an artist is as essential as a scalpel to a surgeon.

I wonder how often we have talked about these tools while we passionately and enthusiastically look for the foundations in a store.

These tools hold the power to create an everyday look, transforming an everyday look into artistry.

Let us discuss the brushes that come in a brush set or sometimes we purchase them as individual brushes.

Each brush has three main parts: the head, ferrule, and handle, each serving a specific purpose.

- **Head:** Soft on the skin, durable, easy to clean.
- **Ferrule:** The metal section holding the bristles.
- **Handle:** Varies in length, chosen based on brush purpose.

Points to keep in mind when purchasing a brush:

- **Purpose:** What product will you use it for?
- **Grip:** The handle should be firm and not too slippery or lightweight.
- **Length:** Choose a length that feels comfortable during use.
- **Bristle Quality:** Look for soft yet resilient bristles that hold their shape.
- **Bristle Density:** Check if it's sparse, dense, or just right based on the application.

Types of brushes:

- **Face Brushes:** Flat brush, round brush, stippling brush, blush brush, contour brush, fan brush.
- **Eye Brushes:** Eye crease (round fluffy brush), shader brush (small, medium, large), blending brush, eyeliner brush, and bent eyeliner brush.
- **Lips and Brows:** Lipstick brush, dual-purpose brow brush, disposable spoolie.

Tips for Using Makeup Tools

- **Layering:** Use brushes and sponges in combination for a polished, blended look. Start with brushes for application and then use a sponge for seamless blending.

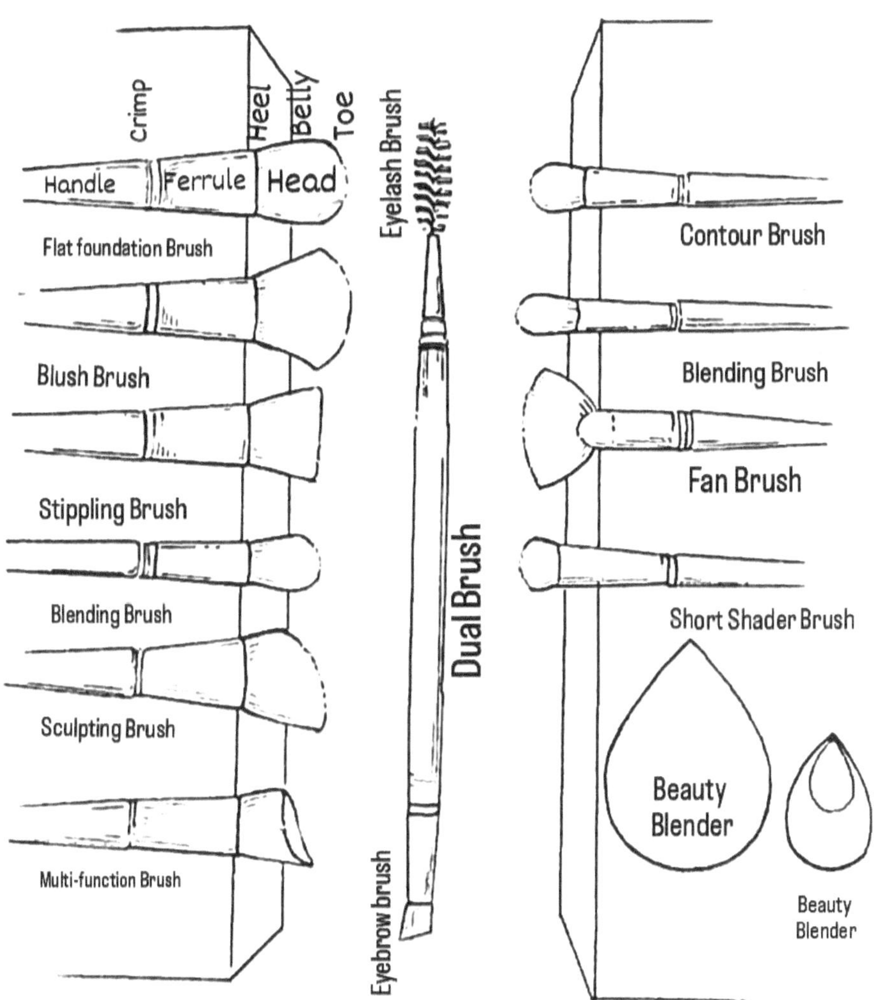

Dry the brushes with the head hanging off the edge
to avoid contact with surface as shown in picture.

- **If a brush drops onto the ground:** Disinfect it before reusing. Ideally, keep it aside and clean it later after finishing your makeup.
- **Product-specific uses:** Flat brushes work best for creams and liquid products, while round brushes are ideal for powders. Whether to use round brushes for cream or liquid products is a personal choice. Spoolie shapes the brows and can even help neaten the hairline during makeup application.

Cleaning the Brushes:

1. **Prepare a gentle solution:** Add a few drops of baby shampoo to water.
2. **Soak:** Dip the brushes just below the ferrule to prevent water from reaching the handle. Let them sit for 10-15 minutes.
3. **Rinse:** Clean each brush individually in fresh water.
4. **Disinfect:** Use a 1:1 mixture of isopropyl alcohol and water (optional).
5. **Dry:** Gently squeeze out excess water, then lay them flat on a soft cloth with the bristles hanging off the edge to avoid contact with the surface, as shown in the picture. I usually leave mine to dry overnight.
6. **Inspect regularly:** Replace brushes that show signs of fraying or have lost shape.

After a couple of uses, makeup brushes accumulate dead cells, dirt, and debris from makeup; therefore, regular cleaning is important to maintain hygiene.

This guide aims to help readers choose and use brushes with confidence. It provides tips to explore different types of tools and shares information that makes each tool a valuable part of your makeup journey. While this guide doesn't cover every brush available on the market, it focuses on helping you select the ones that best suit your preferences and needs.

Watching tutorials can be a helpful starting point to understand how each brush is used. Like any hobby or sport, makeup has a practical learning curve; practice is essential. If you find it challenging to achieve a seamless finish, consider learning under a skilled guide.

I hope my readers find the guidance I once missed during my own makeup journey. Sharing the knowledge that I gained the hard way is my way of serving others on this path.

My Encounter with Brushes

When I first bought my brush set, as per the list I received for purchasing beauty products, I was completely overwhelmed by the number of brushes. I didn't know what to do with any of them except the blush and lipstick brushes. It took time to learn and figure out how to use the angled brush for my eyebrows correctly. As I continued on my learning journey, I developed a preference for certain brushes, and over time, my collection of favourites grew.

One brush that really caught my attention was the fan brush. There's something about its unique look that made it feel fancy. I loved the soft, supple bristles that felt so luxurious against my skin as I used them to highlight my cheekbones. It was a small but joyful moment I truly enjoyed.

As I learned more about each brush and the value it added to my makeup routine, I found it difficult to pick just one favourite. Each brush seemed to have its own importance, its own role in helping me achieve that perfect look. Therefore, it becomes important to learn this craft to use the right tools to create a desired look for oneself.

If I had to choose a favourite, it would be the set I received from Mrs. Lebanon, Rima El Masri, during the International Pageant gift exchange activity. The quality of the brushes was exceptional, and I could feel the thoughtfulness and love that went into choosing them. That set has become my favourite because of the cherished memories associated with it. It is a piece of the journey I have travelled, and I carry it with me everywhere I go. That set is a constant reminder that beauty isn't just what we apply on the outside; it's the energy, the loving relationships, and the fond experiences that stayed with me long after, making it truly magical.

What about you? Do you have a special brush set or makeup tool that holds a meaningful story or memory for you?

CHAPTER ACTIVITY: TOOL TESTING & MASTERY
Part 1: Tool Treasure Hunt

Gather Tools

Collect all your makeup tools, including brushes, sponges, tweezers, eyelash curlers, etc. If you don't have all the tools listed in the chapter, make a note of which ones you're missing.

Part 2: Cleaning Challenge

Brush and Sponge Cleaning Routine

Follow the chapter's cleaning instructions for brushes and sponges. After cleaning, compare the look and feel of each tool before and after.

Reflection

Note how the tool's performance changes after cleaning. For instance, does a freshly cleaned sponge blend foundation more smoothly? Are a brush's bristles softer?

Part 3: Mix and Match Experiment

Objective: Explore the versatility of tools like the palette knife, mixing tray, and sponge.

Create Custom Shades

Mixing different shades of foundation, blush, or cream lipstick on a mixing tray allows you to create personalised colours. Test the blend on your hand or face to check the unique results.

Try Layering

Use a brush for the initial application and a sponge for blending. Layer the products to *make a* difference in the finish.

Quiz: How Well Do You Know Your Tools?

This short quiz will reinforce knowledge about the tools discussed in the chapter.

1. **What is the best way to use a beauty blender for optimal blending?**
   A) Apply foundation directly on the blender when dry
   B) Dampen it first, then squeeze out excess water
   C) Use it with powder products only

2. **Which of the following tools helps create a lifted look for lashes before applying mascara?**
   A) Tweezers
   B) Eyelash Curler
   C) Lip Brush

3. **Why is it important to avoid soaking the ferrule when cleaning brushes?**
   A) It makes the brush slippery
   B) It weakens the bristles
   C) Water can loosen the glue holding the bristles

4. **What's a key benefit of using a mixing tray?**
   A) It avoids direct contact with hands for better hygiene
   B) It helps blend powder products only
   C) It's only useful for professional artists

5. **Which tool should you use if you want a very precise application of lipstick?**
   A) Beauty Blender
   B) Lip Brush
   C) Sponge

6. **What's the main purpose of a spoolie brush?**
   A) Applying foundation evenly
   B) Blending eyeshadow
   C) Shaping brows and separating lashes

7. **How often should you clean your beauty blender or makeup sponge for optimal hygiene?**
   A) Every month
   B) After each use or every few uses
   C) Only when it looks dirty

Correct answers:

| 1 (B) | 2 (B) | 3 (C) | 4 (A) | 5 (B) | 6 (C) | 7 (B) |

Reflect and Journal

What do you think about your experience with the tools you have?

1. Which tool do you feel most comfortable with, and why?
2. Are there any tools that surprised you in terms of effectiveness or ease of use?
3. After completing these activities, which tool would you like to invest in next and why?

These activities and quiz questions will not only deepen your knowledge but also foster a more hands-on understanding of the tools you have or want to acquire. It will help solidify your understanding of why and how each tool is used, allowing you to build confidence gradually.

I wish and hope this book to leave all my readers with newfound skills and confidence.

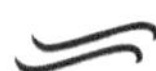

Chapter 15

Everyday Look vs Special Occasions

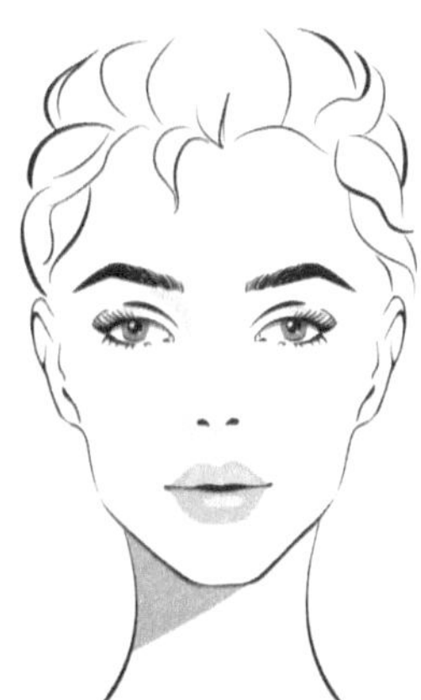

Now that we've explored each product in detail throughout the previous chapters, it's time to put that knowledge to work. This chapter will be a step-by-step guide to creating different looks, from Natural to No-makeup looks to special occasion looks.

If you have read the chapters and completed the activities associated with each chapter, then you are ready to create the look for yourself and enjoy the process. If you haven't read the book and feel that you know your products well, I encourage you to explore. If not, take a moment to read the previous chapters to understand the essentials.

A Step-by-Step Guide

Before we start, here's a reminder from Bhumika Bahl:

'Your makeup is good if your skin is good.'

This quote motivates me to stay committed to my health goals to achieve clean and clear skin.

There is no rule book for makeup. I believe makeup is an art without rules – it's all about finding peace with how you want to present yourself. What others see shapes their perception. The first impression is always visual and leaves an imprint on others.

Having gained a better understanding of our skin and face shape, we are now ready to make informed choices about what products best suit us. Let's start applying these insights to create a look that is perfect for everyday wear.

Natural Look: Effortless and Fresh

This look is great for everyday wear, offering a polished yet subtle appearance.

Key Elements:
- Lightweight Coverage
- Dewy or natural finish.
- Skin like Texture

Steps for a Minimalistic Natural Look:
1. Start with CTMB; give it 3-4 minutes to absorb.
2. Apply sunscreen and give this layer 3-4 minutes to absorb.
3. Dab translucent powder on your face using a soft, fluffy brush. Let it sit for 10 minutes to absorb moisture for a long-lasting, smooth finish.
4. Use a soft brown monochrome for eyes (optional).
5. Define the brows.
6. Finish it off using kohl (optional), eyeliner (optional), and mascara (colourless mascara - optional)
7. Apply lipstick. Define your lips well using a pencil, fill the lips with cream, and top it up with liquid lipstick before adding a little shine with lip gloss (optional). My lips are never complete without lip gloss.
8. Remove excess powder from the face and blend it well using a round fluffy brush or a beauty blender.
9. Apply powder blush for a matte finish.
10. Add soft strokes of highlighter to add a little sparkle (optional). My makeup is never complete without this step.
11. Spritz your face generously with setting spray or fixing spray for a flawless, long-lasting finish.

> Tip: Take a moment to ensure each layer has been absorbed; your patience will make all the difference for a natural, long-lasting look.

Natural Look: 'No-Makeup' Makeup Look

- **Medium Coverage**
- **Long-Wear Finish**
- **Highlight optional**

Steps for 'No-Makeup' Makeup Look:

1. Start with CTMBP. People whose skin has pores or certain flaws that make them uncomfortable can add primer according to their skin type for a smoother surface.
2. Apply colour corrector to hide dark circles, blemishes, or uneven skin tone.
3. Apply concealer to create a uniform skin tone.
4. A well-blended soft layer of foundation for a seamless finish.
5. Dab translucent powder on your face using a soft, fluffy brush. Let it sit for 10 minutes to absorb moisture for a long-lasting, smooth finish.
6. Spritz setting spray for the layers to settle.
7. Use a soft brown or any preferred monochrome for the eyes.
8. Define the brows.
9. Finish it off with kajal (optional), eyeliner (optional), and mascara (colourless—optional).
10. Apply lipstick. Define your lips well using a pencil, fill the lips with cream, and top it up with liquid lipstick before adding a little shine with lip gloss (optional).
11. Remove extra powder from the face and blend it well using a round fluffy brush or a beauty blender. This step gives me the confidence to carry a polished look throughout the day.
12. Contour your face to add depth. Use cream or liquid contour for a dewy look; use powder for a matte finish.
13. Apply liquid or cream blush for a dewy look or use powder blush for a matte finish.
14. Add soft strokes of highlighter to add a little sparkle (optional).
15. Spritz your face generously with setting spray or fixing spray for a flawless, long-lasting finish.

> Tip: Ensure each layer dries before applying the next layer. Your patience will make all the difference for a natural, long-lasting look. You can use a small hand fan to quicken the drying process.

Self-Reflection:

How do you feel when you wear this natural look? Do you feel fresh and confident, or do you prefer to add more for a different effect?

Every day is a chance to feel fresh and naturally you. Remember, patience and practice are the key, and soon you'll find each step as easy as picking your favourite lipstick!

Now that we've practised the everyday natural looks, let's take things up a notch for those special occasions where you want to shine a little brighter. The glam look is designed for long-lasting wear, with added coverage and dimension.

Glam Look: Flawless and Long-Lasting

To create a look for special occasions:

Key Elements:

- Full Coverage
- Long-Wear Finish
- Dimensional Contour and Highlight

Steps for a Glam Look:

- Step 1: Skin Preparation: Start with CTMBP. Prime your skin to smooth out texture and create a base for your foundation.
- Step 2: Colour Corrector.
- Step 3: Colour Concealer.
- Step 4: Foundation Choice: Opt for full coverage with a matte or dewy finish to create a flawless base that lasts throughout the extended event all day long. Use a brush to apply the foundation, blending with gentle tapping motions for an even finish. Always start from the centre of your face and blend outward. Cover all areas evenly. Build up the foundation in layers if you need extra correction.
- Step 5: Use Setting Spray.
- Step 6: Highlight the seven points on the face using a lighter shade; blend well using a beauty blender.
- Step 7: Dab translucent powder generously on the highlighted areas. This technique is called baking, and it works exceptionally well for me before

doing my eye makeup. It also helps keep fine lines at bay by providing a long-lasting smooth finish.

- Step 8: Complete your eye makeup with or without using shimmers or glitters and false eyelashes. Using coloured eyeliners and coloured mascara is a personal choice.
- Step 9: Apply lipstick.
- Step 10: Dust off any extra translucent powder from the face and blend well for a smooth finish.
- Step 11: Contour using liquid or powder and blend it well to give your face a well-sculpted illusion.
- Step 12: Blush, liquid, or cream is a personal choice. Remember to lock it with powder using the same colour.
- Step 13: Finishing touches with bronzing and highlighting.
- Step 14: Define your lips and add a little shine using lip gloss for a perfect pout.

Self-Reflection

- What is your favourite part of the glam process?
- Does it make you feel powerful, elegant, or creative? Why?

Before you start applying makeup, it is important to have a blueprint for the look you want to create. To get inspired, browse online for looks you connect with, such as natural, classic, or glamorous. Choose pictures from the internet or magazines that align with your style and personality.

Once you have the pictures in front of you, it will be easier for you to understand your taste, style, and the techniques and products you require to achieve that goal.

By following these guidelines, readers can confidently enhance their look—whether subtle, natural, or glam. Having the right products, learning the right techniques, and practising are key.

Makeup techniques and products have evolved tremendously over time, and they will continue to do so. The question is, are we evolving with them? Are we ready to embrace change to narrow the gap with Generation Alpha?

Staying current is a powerful choice that can boost your confidence and enrich your knowledge so that you can stay connected meaningfully with younger generations.

Whether we want to use the knowledge—or not; it's a personal choice—but staying updated and upgrading yourself in the fields of your choice should be a conscious choice to live a happy life filled with purpose.

I hope this chapter serves as a useful guide, just as it has guided me, especially for those looking to build confidence in makeup application. The structured approach has helped me take one step at a time, making the process feel manageable.

Now that you have the tools and knowledge, take your time, enjoy the process, and create a look that feels uniquely you.

On this beautiful Diwali morning in 2024, I find myself reflecting on my journey. My daughter, a dedicated doctor, has gone to the hospital for her duty, leaving me in the peaceful embrace of her home in Chennai. As I look through the French window into the open sky, I feel a deep connection with nature, refreshing my spirit and inspiring me to return to my work after a short break. Just as the festival of Diwali brings light to the darkest night, our makeup has the power to hide the flaws that make us uncomfortable while highlighting our best features and illuminating the beauty within. Whether it's a subtle natural look or a bold glam look, each one reflects who we are at that moment.

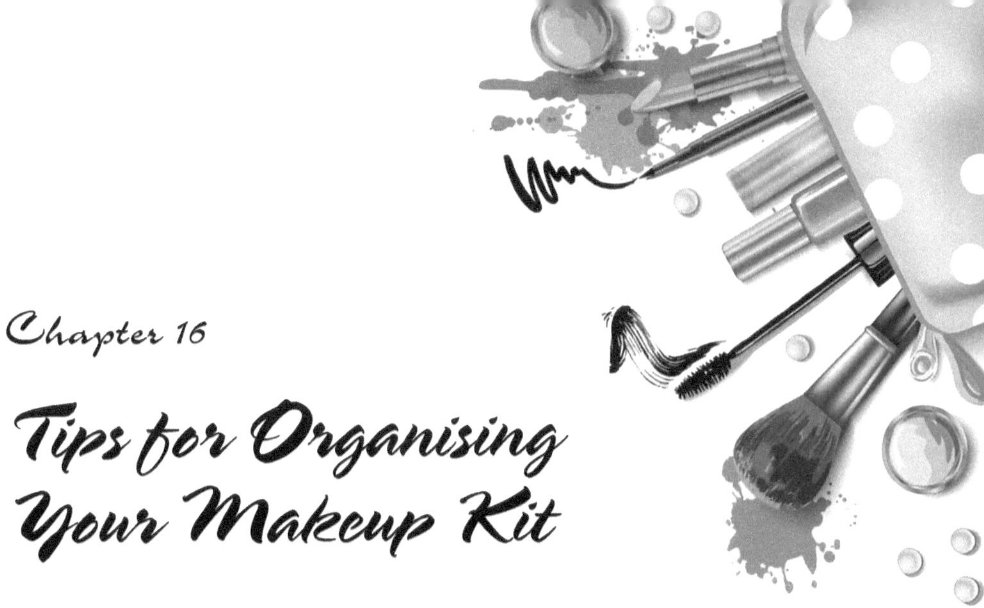

Chapter 16

Tips for Organising Your Makeup Kit

As I write this chapter, I reflect on the motivation that has driven me to write this book. My journey has been filled with trials and errors. It was at the age of 50+, only through organised and structured training that I finally began to fit the jigsaw puzzle of makeup knowledge together. In the beginning, the overwhelming array of products left me confused. My purchasing decisions were often influenced by opinions from others who weren't experts themselves, whether it was friends, online influencers, or salespeople behind counters.

Now that I understand the various products and their uses, I make informed choices based on my own knowledge and experience. This is why I have chosen not to name specific brands in this book. Makeup is deeply personal, and each individual's choices depend on several factors: budget, the desire to experiment with trends versus sticking to conventional products, preference for domestic versus international brands, and whether one leans towards natural, herbal, or commercial options.

Here's a well-structured list of essential products that one should have in their vanity, organised into categories for better clarity:

Essential Products for Your Vanity

Skincare Essentials

1 Cleanser

2 Toner

3 Moisturiser

4 Beauty Oils or Serums

Makeup Base

5 Primer

6 Colour Corrector (liquid, cream)

7 Concealer (liquid, cream)

8 Foundation (liquid, cream)

9 Loose Powder or Pressed Powder

10 Skin Illuminator

11 Highlighter (liquid, powder)

12 Contour (liquid, cream, powder)

13 Bronzer (powder)

14 Blush (liquid, cream, powder)

Eye Makeup

15 Eyebrow Gel

16 Eyebrow Wax

17 Eyeshadows (powder)

18 Shimmer, Glitters, or Lid Frost

19 Kohl

20 Eyeliner (liquid or cream)

21 Fake Eyelashes (optional)

22 Coloured Lenses (optional)

23 Mascara (Black, Coloured, Transparent)

Lip Products
24 Lip Balm
25 Lip Liner
26 Cream Lipstick
27 Liquid Lipstick
28 Lip Gloss or Lip Plumper

Finishing Touches
29 Setting Spray
30 Finishing Spray
31 Makeup Remover

Tools
32 Mixing Plate with Palette Knife
33 Beauty Blenders
34 Tweezers (optional)
35 Makeup Brushes

Miscellaneous
Earbuds
Cotton Swabs
Wet Wipes
Face Wipes
Sanitiser
Hand fan

This comprehensive list offers a foundation of 31 essentials, but feel free to personalise it by selecting products that resonate with your style. Whether you are a beginner or an enthusiast, it ensures you have everything needed to create a variety of looks while keeping your vanity organised. Remember to handle your products with love and care, and always keep your tools clean to maintain their longevity.

Now that you have your essentials in place, let's move on to a few practical tips for keeping your makeup kit organised and well-maintained.

A Few Tips

Declutter Regularly

- Review Expiry Dates: Regularly check the expiry dates on your products.
- Assess Usage: consider donating or discarding those products that have been sitting unused for a couple of months.

Categorise Your Products

- *By Type*: Organise your makeup into categories, making finding easy
- *By Frequency of Use*: Place your most-used products within easy reach while storing less frequently used items further away.

Storage Solution

- Makeup Bags and Organisers: Use clear containers with compartments to easily spot your products.
- Drawer Organisers: Keep everything neat and tidy with drawer organisers.

Labelling

- Use Labels: If you have a larger collection, labelling can help you locate products quickly.
- Clean Your Makeup Tools: Regular cleaning and sanitising of makeup brushes and sponges is essential to maintaining hygiene and extending their longevity.
- Storage for Brushes: Keep your brushes upright and organised. I use a makeup brush pouch, which is handy and easy to use.

Final Thoughts

"A tidy makeup kit makes your daily routine easier, fuelling creativity and helping you confidently enhance your natural beauty every day."

Travel-Friendly Essentials – Packing Smart

As a pageant girl, packing light was one of the biggest challenges. If you're travelling overseas by economy with a 15kg limit, makeup can easily take up half the space and weight in your bag. I am sure anyone who's been through this journey would agree! It took me quite some time to get my essentials right. I tend to pack a little extra, just in case, but here is a list of the minimum essentials for a polished look for beginners to travel light.

A Guide to Travel-Friendly Essentials and Packing Smart:

Multi-Use Makeup Products

- *BB Cream or Tinted Moisturiser*: Perfect for a natural look without worrying about foundation.
- *Lip and Cheek Tint*: Personally, I often use my lipstick as a blush, which works great while travelling. A small cream palette is a good idea. It can be used for eyeshadow as well.
- *Cream or Powder Eyeshadow Palette*: I carry a small powder palette of neutral shades, which works well for both morning and evening looks.
- *Kajal, Eyeliner, Mascara*: While I can skip kajal and eyeliner, if necessary, mascara is a must to complete my eye makeup.

Compact Skincare

- Travel-Sized Cleansing Wipes: Perfect for quick cleanses on the go.
- CTM Products: Opt for sample-sized cleansers, toners, and moisturisers. Some brands offer travel sets, or you can decant your favourite products to keep things light.

Accessories and Tools

- Multifunctional Brush: A dual-ended brush or versatile flat and round brushes minimise the number you would want to carry. Look for brushes that work for both eyes and face makeup.
- Makeup Remover Wipes: Regular wet wipes are also great for travel, keeping things lightweight.

Travel Considerations

- Compact Makeup Bags: Choose a lightweight, see-through, spill-proof bag with compartments or sections to organise essentials.
- Sample Sizes: Carry sample-sized products for easy packing that fit easily in your luggage.

- Prioritise Versatility: Go for products with multiple uses, such as a lip tint that doubles as blush.
- Stay Organised: Keep essentials in a designated pouch to easily access them and quickly find what you need.

By packing multifunctional products, you can travel light and still look polished. A minimal makeup approach works best for travel, allowing you to look your best without the bulk.

Organising your makeup kit not only keeps it looking neat and visually appealing but also transforms your space into a daily retreat. It's a space that prepares you to put your best foot forward every day, your place of happiness and creativity, your personal sanctuary.

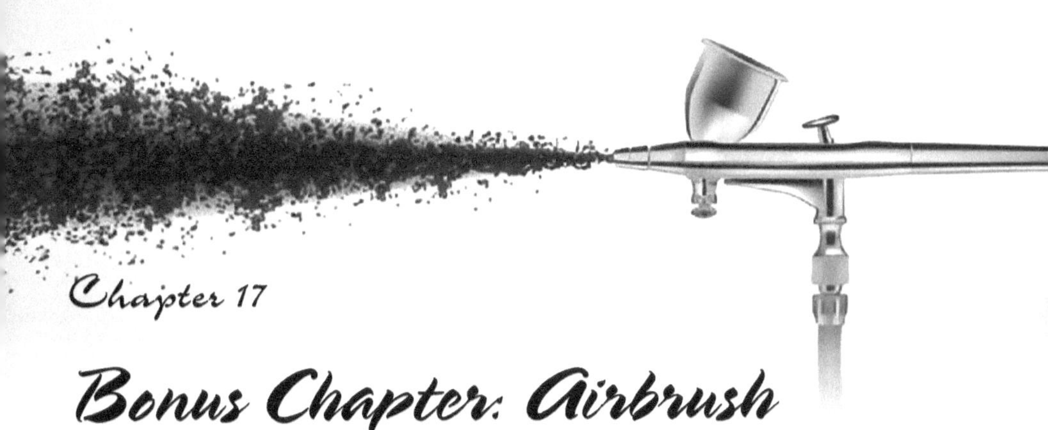

Chapter 17

Bonus Chapter: Airbrush

Makeup truly is an art—a balance of precision, patience, and building layer by layer. I used to think lipstick was simple; you just swipe it on, maybe change the colour for variety. But when I began learning about makeup, I discovered that even something as familiar as lipstick has layers of skill. Prepping the lips so the colour glides on smoothly, using techniques to extend its staying power, each small step transforms how the lipstick feels, looks, and lasts. I never realised how many secrets were hidden in plain sight!

People rarely share these tips openly. Sure, there are exceptions, but in my experience, so much of makeup artistry feels like a well-guarded treasure. I could see this clearly as I explored different techniques and practised things like blurring edges with a sponge or brush. Even a small technique, like softening the lines for a natural finish, is surprisingly intricate. With enough practice, it becomes second nature, a kind of muscle memory—effortless but only because of hours spent perfecting it.

My curiosity led me to formal training, not just for tips and tricks but to deeply understand each step. Through trial and error and a few scattered lessons, I picked up bits of knowledge, but I wanted to take it further. When I joined Bhumika Bahl's academy, I felt like I stepped into a whole new world. One of the most exciting things I learned there was the airbrush technique. I had been working with makeup for over a year and a half, and until then, no one had mentioned it! It was such an intriguing concept that it immediately sparked my curiosity.

I didn't train to become a makeup artist for others; I trained to be better for myself. In pageants, makeup is an essential skill—a way to express and empower oneself on stage. But there's another reason: my daughter. I wanted to keep learning. Over the years, experimenting with makeup together has been our bonding ritual. Now, as she grows into her own style, I feel even more inspired to improve my skills. I love that makeup brings us both so much joy, creating little moments of art together. Through this journey, makeup has become more than just a skill. She inspires me to keep evolving. It's a way to connect, express, and grow—not just for pageants but for life.

Airbrush Makeup: A Leap Forward in Cosmetic Application

My fondness for an airbrush machine grew due to the flawless finish it provides and the luxurious feel it leaves on the skin. I learned to work with a gravity-feed, dual-action airbrush gun, which has proven to be both effective and enjoyable.

The Airbrush System: 3 Main Components

1. **Compressor**: The compressor draws in air, compresses it, and directs the compressed air through the airbrush. A moisture control filter (MCF) prevents any atmospheric moisture from passing into the airbrush gun, ensuring a smooth application.

2. **Dual-Action Airbrush Gun**: This type of gun allows for precise control over air pressure and product flow with the use of a trigger, making it easier to adjust coverage and achieve a seamless finish.

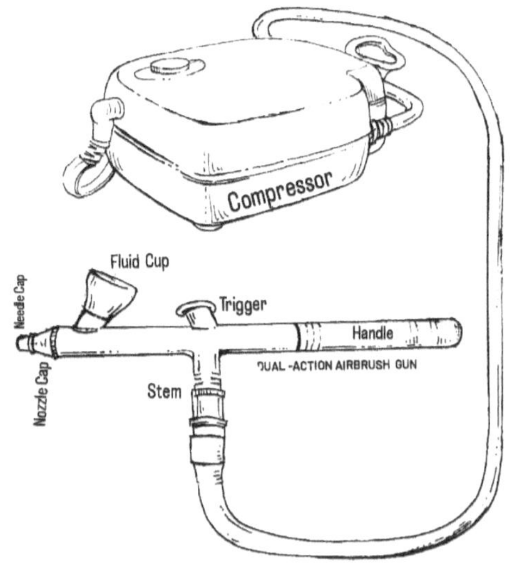

3. **Makeup Products**: Liquid makeup products with dropper dispensers are specially formulated for use with airbrush systems, allowing smooth and even application.

How Airbrush Makeup Differs from Regular Makeup

1. **Hygienic Application**: Airbrush makeup is applied without direct contact with brushes or sponges, making it a more hygienic option.
2. **Luxurious Experience**: Each spritz feels refreshing, almost like a mini spa experience.
3. **Seamless Finish**: It provides a sheer, smooth finish with evenly diffused pigment, avoiding any visible lines.
4. **Buildable Coverage**: Layers can be built up gradually without feeling heavy on the skin.
5. **Long-Lasting Results**: The makeup has a flawless finish that lasts throughout the day.
6. **Minimal Touch-Ups**: It sets well on the skin, reducing the need for touch-ups.
7. **Product Efficiency**: A small amount of product delivers excellent results.
8. **Customizable**: Some airbrush systems allow you to mix your favourite products with a makeup solution to achieve the correct consistency.
9. **Convenience**: The system is easy to use and easy to clean.

What I Love About Airbrush Makeup

It offers less hassle, fewer products, and a flawless, long-lasting finish. It's my go-to for my morning and evening CTM routine. A sheer foundation and a touch of blush give me a perfect look.

Downsides of Using Airbrush Makeup

1. **Initial Investment**: Purchasing a quality kit can be costly.
2. **Skill Requirement**: Mastering the technique requires practice, ideally under guidance from a skilled mentor.

3. **Product Availability**: Airbrush products are not as readily available as traditional makeup.

4. **Power Dependency**: The system requires a power source to operate.

5. **Touch-Ups**: Not ideal for quick touch-ups; once applied, touch-ups generally require traditional tools.

6. **Limited for Eye and Lip Makeup**: For detailed eye makeup and lipstick, I find traditional application methods are more useful.

One Drawback When Using an Airbrush on Oneself

When working on oneself, there's a chance of product particles getting into the eyes since the makeup is sprayed from a distance and feels very light on the skin. Over time, this could potentially affect eye health. However, it's safe when applied by a skilled hand to someone else, as the eyes remain closed during application.

Steps I Follow When Using the Airbrush Gun

1. **Cleansing**
2. **Toning**
3. **Moisturising**
4. **Priming:** For self-application, I prefer using a regular primer to ensure the safety of my eyes. However, if someone else is doing my makeup, I enjoy using a liquid primer for its smooth finish.
5. **Foundation**
6. **Contour**
7. **Blush**
8. **Highlighter** to finish the look

I use this technique for a minimal makeup look or a "no-makeup" makeup look. I love the fresh, natural finish it creates. For me, the airbrush technique offered a fresh perspective on the beauty in each layer.

My Advice on Makeup

My advice for anyone interested in makeup is to learn the craft under a skilled trainer to understand the techniques thoroughly. I am a certified makeup artist from Bhumika Bahl's academy and a Certified International Airbrush Makeup Artist. I have always believed that skill comes from practice; hours spent perfecting each step truly refine your art.

As I look back at my own makeup journey, I realise that it's more than just the products or techniques; it's about the confidence, artistry, and empowerment that comes with it. Whether you're perfecting a minimal makeup look or experimenting with airbrush techniques, remember this: *makeup is not just about the way you look but how it makes you feel.* Keep exploring, keep learning, and most importantly, keep celebrating your unique self.

Final Activity

Create a community to share and discuss makeup with friends. Why not dedicate one kitty party to exploring foundations and another to diving into the world of blushes? Or turn a coffee date with your girlfriends into a fun conversation about mascaras and eyeliners.

For an extra special twist, plan a mother-daughter makeup session! Take turns adorning each other, embracing the choices you both make and creating cherished memories. Through my own experience, I can tell you how meaningful this can be. This December, my daughter insisted we dress up formally for New Year's Eve. I did my makeup and gave her a glamorous look. She loved it and complimented me on how much better I had become at the craft. It was the first time I wore a gown for New Year's Eve, and both of us received countless compliments that made us smile and giggle. I am so grateful to her for making the eve of 2025 truly special and memorable. This is one of my favourite ways to spend time with my daughter. It's not just about makeup but about bonding and celebrating our unique styles together.

Sharing your makeup journey with friends and family can deepen connections, just as I have found joy in my own bond with my daughter.

Thank you for joining me on this journey. I hope the lessons I have shared, both in technique and in heart, help you create the beauty you've always wanted, inside and out. Stay true to yourself, and let your makeup be a reflection of that inner confidence.

I wish you all the best!
Have fun, look your best every day, and keep your creative juices flowing.
Let your creativity shine through!

About the Author

Amita Goel is a National Beauty Pageant winner whose transformative journey began at age 52. She was crowned **Elite Queen Of The World India 2023-2024**, earning the honour of representing India on the global stage in New York in April 2024, where she achieved the prestigious title of **First Runner-Up at Elite Queen Of The World**.

After more than 30 years as a homemaker, stepping into the world of pageantry reignited her love for makeup, not just as an art form but as a powerful means of self-expression. She had the opportunity to walk in fashion shows, not only as a fashion model but also as a role model, breaking stereotypes. Along the way, she embraced a medicine-free, healthy lifestyle and became a certified makeup artist and an International Airbrush Makeup Artist, proving that reinvention is possible at any age.

With this book, Amita steps into a new role as an author seeking to inspire homemakers, especially those over 50, and the next generation to view makeup as a tool for building confidence, finding one's voice, and celebrating individuality. Her journey, from fumbling with makeup brushes during her pageant training to mastering advanced techniques, demonstrates that it's never too late to chase your dreams.

Amita's writing shines with warmth, relatability, and encouragement. Through practical tips and empowering reflections, she aims to guide the reader through the vibrant world of makeup, inspiring them to embrace their unique style and feel confident at every stage of life.

www.ingramcontent.com/pod-product-compliance
Lightning Source LLC
Chambersburg PA
CBHW031149130726
47988CB00006B/2596